MW01173531

Praise for
A Wise Old Girl's Own Almanac

"From her crystalline memories of childhood to the
humorous vagaries of old age, Joyce Harries finds the
unique in the every day. With the touch of a poet and
the eye of a storyteller, Joyce invites the reader on an
odyssey of a life lived with exuberance."

—Marion Brooker, author of picture book "Tadeo's Search For
Circles" Fitzhenry and Whiteside IPPY gold medal winner 2012; "Hold
The Oxo!" A Teenage Soldier Writes Home, Dundurn Press 2011

"In a cultural climate that inundates us with sound
bites of information, leaving us emotionally, intellectu-
ally, and spiritually undernourished, *A Wise Old Girl's
Own Almanac* offers a smorgasbord of poetry, recipes,
short stories, and personal remembrances that satisfies
and delights. With gentle and straightforward wit,
author Joyce Harries skillfully sifts and kneads through
her pantry of memories, wordplay, and observations
with a balanced combination of wistfulness, pragma-
tism, and optimism."

Renée Layberry, Editor

ISBN
978-1-4602-1439-8 (Hardcover)
978-1-4602-1440-4 (Paperback)
978-1-4602-1441-1 (eBook)

Produced by:

FriesenPress

Suite 300 — 852 Fort Street
Victoria, BC, Canada V8W 1H8

www.friesenpress.com

Distributed to the trade by The Ingram Book Company

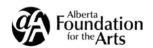

A Wise Old Girl's Own Almanac

MEMOIRS, FICTION, ESSAYS, RECIPES AND POETRY

by Joyce Harries

Illustrated by Tasli Shaw

To: Pat

Best wishes —

Joyce Harries

2014

Books by Joyce Harries

Girdles and Other Harnesses I Have Known

Twice in a Blue Moon

A Wise Old Girl's Own Almanac

Dedication

For my children, Bruce and wife Karen, Jody, Lori, Jeffrey
and wife Noni, and Daniel. For my grandchildren: Bill
vanEgteren and partner Jessie Macdonald, Stephanie Harries
and partner Jesse Meyer, and Lucas Harries, Tommy Wilson
and partner Hannah McNeice, Lori and Annie Wilson, Tasli
and Kyli Shaw, Molly, Hu, Rosie, Katie, Angus, Maggie, Bruce,
Emmett and Annie Harries and for my great grandchild
Owen vanEgteren. Especially remembering my husband
Hu, son Tommy and my parents, Bruce and Ethel Farrell.

Foreword

A Wise Old Girls' Own Almanac is the same only different from my first book, *Girdles and Other Harnesses I Have Known*. This time there's more fiction and it too is definitely "made up". It seems I can't only write about me and mine and what I think about - all those sweet and sour reminders that life is good.

Table of Contents

* denotes story also appears in Athabasca
University's Alberta Women's Memory Project

They Say, I Say

they say
cut to the chase
shorten your stories
I say
I'm trying
to share an experience
why must I boil it down
to its essence
deglaze it
evaporate it
to an extract
what will we talk about
in the spaces
around the words
you say
I should leave out
please
relax
listen
slide into reverie
linger with me

Joyce Harries, 1928 –

Choices

"Quaint." That's what young people might say today. Well, no, they wouldn't say "quaint", they'd say, "weird — but why didn't you just *go?*"

Here's how it was: It was nineteen forty-six, before I was in the picture, and Hu had been awarded an Imperial Order Daughters of the Empire fellowship to study for a Ph.D. at the London School of Economics. He'd had the date deferred a year because of some economic studies he was doing for the Executive Council of the provincial government and he'd also stepped in to teach for a sick professor at the university.

We met in the fall of forty-seven. A blind date that blossomed into forever love before Christmas. Then in the spring of forty-eight, when he reapplied for the fellowship we had become engaged, and were making wedding plans for August.

When Hu tried to get the stipulation of "award to single status recipients only" waived for "married status", the I.O.D.E. wouldn't bend. Regretfully, he gave up his longed-for opportunity. He was twenty-six and I was nineteen. Looking back, I shake my head thinking how absolutely naive and ignorant I was of such matters. I truly did not understand the choice Hu had made. Why didn't I just go overseas with him? The idea never occurred to me and he never asked. Remember, times were different. Attending L.S.E. for a doctorate was an incredible opportunity for a scholar like Hu. Oh dear. Years later, I found letters from his mother written at that time. She had folded into the letter a Calgary newspaper clipping showing a gowned Hu with a caption: "Local man receives fellowship to London School of Economics." We would have lived in peacetime London with its post-war shortages, and I would have grown up sooner. What would it have done for Hu's future? Perhaps he would have stayed in academia.

If the choice presented itself to a child of ours, though of course "single only" hadn't been a fellowship funding criterion for years, I would say, "Wait a year to be married." or more likely, "Go for it — live in sin or live there not in sin."

Of course, our life without L.S.E. turned out quite satisfactorily. We married and had six children. Hu taught at the University and completed his Ph.D. at the University in the States, where he had earned one of his Master's degrees, but this was the difficult path. With his studies complete, Hu worked as an economist. He started his own small consulting firm and began dabbling in the entrepreneurial world he would remain in for the rest of our life together. And then there was the world of politics. Another choice.

I guess one can look back, not with regrets, but with wonder at choices made, opportunities taken and lost. Funny isn't it? Guess that's what life's all about: choices. But what makes us make the choices we do?

> *There is neither vice nor virtue, there are*
> *only circumstances.* — Balzac

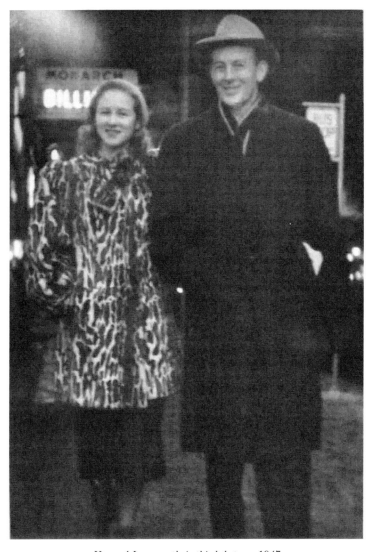

Hu and Joyce on their third date — 1947

Sex and Money*

You'd think by now, at my age, I'd be better at it. Not sex, which once I was, though now I'm out of practice, but money, because when I was young we had very little of it.

I don't recall ever pining for anything to the extent that I pleaded, except for a baby brother or sister. This request involved both money and sex, in which I never dreamed my parents indulged. My parents never spoke of either money or sex in my presence, even when I found condoms in my father's sock drawer. What was I doing in there anyway? And I told my cousin and he told my aunt and she told my mother and my mother told me, "Never mind what they are. It's private and keep out of our drawers." My dad wasn't present for this pronouncement.

When I think of my parents' planned parenthood stance, I know their decision to have only one child had a lot to do with money, or the lack thereof. They both knew, coming from large families, in my father's — nine children, in my mother's — six, how hard it would be in depression times. They must have resolved they would have more time and wherewithal for one child than for a flock. I was born in 1928.

I don't think I got allowances until I was six, and then it was five cents a week. The allowance wasn't for school supplies. I would spend it on jaw-breakers or hideous wax pink and white false teeth, which disintegrated into flaky bits and stuck to the roof of my mouth. I don't recall my parents ever paying me to do odd jobs or deduct from my allowance because I didn't make my bed or hang up my pajamas or get all A's on my report card (which is fortunate because I rarely did.) We didn't pay *our* children for good marks or for promising not to smoke before they were twenty-one. I sometimes think these bribes would have been a good idea, after watching neighbors' success in this field.

When I was a child I would be sent to the Red and White store for a loaf of bread or half a pound of bacon, but was not given money since we ran a tab. Years later, I found at the back of one of my mother's cookbooks, in her beautiful script, small wavering lines of expenses from January 1928. eight months before my birth. She had noted her budget for the first week of that month as "$3.00." When I was fifteen months old, in November 1929, her monthly total budget was $50.00. What I now know, but didn't know then, was not only did they have difficulty paying the rent on their little pink bungalow, they likely had trouble paying the Red and White grocery bill too.

When I was older, and visited my Aunt Ruby who worked in the millinery department of Johnston Walkers, she would take a grubby change purse with a metal squeeze-twist closing out of her long black double-handled bag. From it she would extract a quarter with a picture of King George the fifth on it and tell me to "buy treats or go to a show." Then the change purse would snap shut, and she would plop it back into the depths of her bag. A small cloud of pale pink powder would puff onto the front of her black crepe dress. I would thank her, and rush off to spend the rare quarter as fast as I could.

> *A cynic knows the price of everything and the value of nothing.* — Oscar Wilde

*The above story can also be found in Athabasca University's Alberta Women's Memory Project under "Memoir Collection".

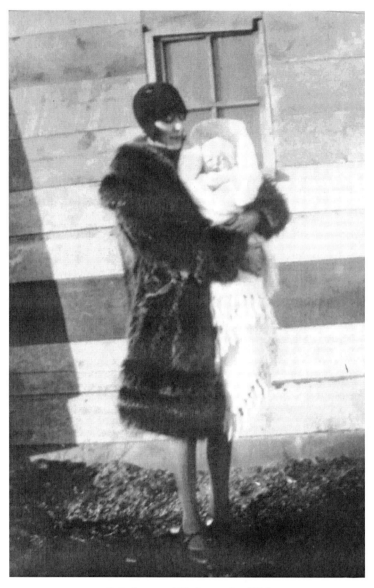

Baby Joyce and Mother — Oct 1928

The King is Dead

mother said
gumboots aren't good for your eyes
I wonder why she always had
odd excuses for the forbidden
don't make a funny face
it might stick that way
no you can't wear knee socks yet
you'll get a chill in your bladder
and why couldn't I have
worn the navy bloomers with knee socks
instead of the long tan colored
stockings held up with garters
attached to a white cotton waist
only the knees and five inches
of skin would get cold

boys had gumboots
with orange rubber soles and tops
lucky girls had
thin rubber boots
shiny black when new
then dull after full dunkings

the pond had tiny bugs that
could walk on water
they could
skittered as though
the surface was glass
Jackie launched a boat
with a wind- up prop
that tangled in weeds
water over the top of his gumboots

and we built a raft with old boards
behind the Becker's garage
my dad said
to be safe
let me try it
he wore Packard maroon leather
bedroom slippers
as he stepped on our craft
it tilted to starboard
hit a shoal
sank beneath the briny
we didn't know whether
to laugh or cry
but my dad said
that was lucky
no one drowned

and we saw jelly masses
with little black dots
that turned into pollywogs
that turned into frogs
and we caught the frogs
in jars lids punched with nails
took them to Julian's

garden pond
where he played scientist
next to his father's aviary
and his brother's rabbit hutch

it got cold
the pond froze
rubber ice heaved
like a water bed
we slid
water bubbled up in places
then froze
while the raft slept in its depths
it snowed
snowed for days and nights
and we brought toboggans
and sleighs and slid down the hill
across the hidden pond
the street lights shone above
then an older sister came
and said dinner's ready
you have to come home
the King is dead
and she was crying
and I said
who
the King of England
King George the Fifth

I didn't cry
thought
too bad
and took another turn

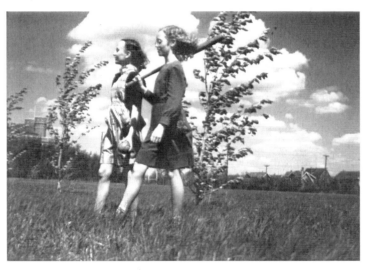

Joyce and Daurel in field across from home — 1937

Christmas Oranges

When I was growing up in the Thirties and when my children were young in the Fifties small Christmas oranges came, as they still do, wrapped individually in orange tissue. Back then they were packed in small lightweight wooden crates, not bright cardboard boxes, and they were called Jap oranges. As a child, I thought it was one word — "Japoranges."

An orange was always in the toe of a Christmas stocking and more sat in a black glass bowl with whole walnuts, pecans and brazil nuts, which were called "nigger toes!" Thankfully these racist expressions have not been used for many years, but I mention them to show that the world has improved in at least a small way.

The oranges smelled the same then as they do today. They too were sweet and the white membrane threads peeled off just as readily. A bad orange would squish blue-green and powdery at the bottom of the box, soaking its tissue protection and smelling rotten just as it happens today.

M.F.K. Fisher wrote of that tiny, special, oh-so-tender section in some oranges and how she would dry these on a windowsill, claiming the insides, encased in a fragile shell, were prizes. I think she was deluded. She would have missed that special orange perfume when she bit into the crystallized pieces and the fine spray in the eye when a section was pierced if separated from its mate. Her morsel would be chewy and not easily swallowed.

There were different ways of going about eating a Christmas orange. Some children quickly gobbled one section after another while the more contemplative ones sucked and savored the orange. Those were the children who examined a parcel by shaking, weighing, and guessing at its contents before finally opening the present. The frenzied ones pounced, tore open and touched the gift, while the contemplative ones were still evaluating the wrapping paper.

Children were taught to peel the orange and put the fragrant peel pieces into the flattened tissue on their laps, finally placing the membrane threads on the top of the pile. Each section was eaten as it was pulled from the whole. The small soft package of pith and rind was then bundled together and thrown in the fireplace. As it burned with pieces of the wooden crate and wrapping paper, the house took on some of our favorite Christmas scents. If the orange wrappings didn't make it into the fireplace, the package would be hidden behind a cushion or under a couch to be found weeks later as hard bits of darkened, wrinkled, cardboard-like specimens even cats or dogs would have no interest in.

Now, the end of the crop of Christmas oranges from the Orient sit in stores until well after the New Year, the fruit not at its perfect peak. More orange globes will turn to blue-green squish.

Then real Christmas trees will be mulched, there will only be turkey soup left in the freezer, cranberry sauce stains will be bleached away, only a small chunk of Christmas cake will remain and not even a crumb of shortbread will be left in the special red Christmas cookie tin. By the time they stop selling Christmas oranges this year, children's digestive systems will have grown accustomed to Florida orange juice and winter bananas once again; their noses and heads will not long for the pine, ginger and orange aromas of Christmas, and neither will I.

> *I'm happy and content because I think I am.*
> — Lesage, Hitoire de Gil Blas, 1735

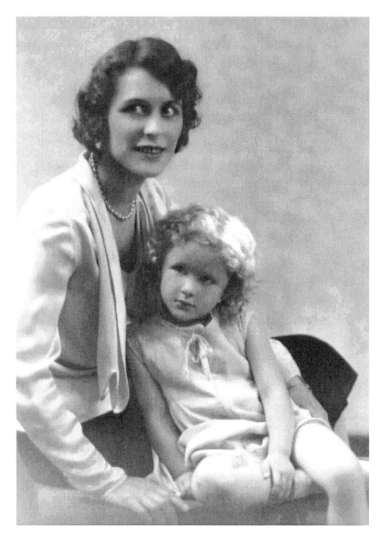

Mother and me — 1931

My Mother and Beauty

Beauty was not a disturbing category for me when I was young. I now recognize that my mother was a beauty teacher by example. She napped briefly most afternoons calling it her *beauty sleep.* This was in the Thirties and it never occurred to me to see if she had changed in any way when she emerged from my parents' bedroom. She would wipe off the Ponds cold cream, pinch her cheeks, squeeze her eyebrows into tidy arches, push back her cuticles and do her dark brown curly hair after dipping her comb under the tap. The final touch was to put on stockings. She would twist sideways, looking down and back, in order to straighten her seams. Then she would sit on the cane-bottomed stool in front of the dresser with the three-paneled mirrors, checking her profile and the back of her head.

Sometimes Mother and I would go for a walk or make cookies. On the days when she skipped her beauty sleep, we would take the streetcar over the high level bridge. We stayed on the streetcar all the way down Jasper Avenue to 101st Street where it turned northeast. We continued, ending up past Borden Park where the streetcar tracks bordered a buffalo paddock. We would get off at 66th Street and walk past summer gardens of sweet William, peonies and nasturtiums on the boardwalk, which was raised in places over willow-ringed ponds.

Mother's family home and garden was our destination. A narrow board-sidewalk went from my grandparents back porch across the lawn and over clumps of frothing baby's breath through a hedge, to my Aunt Elsie and Uncle Billy's back door.

Aunt Elsie was the eldest daughter in the English immigrant family of six daughters. She was blond, fair-skinned, blue-eyed, hard of hearing much of her life, and was the least stylish of my mother's sisters. The next lived three blocks away. Doris: brunette, dark skin and dark-eyed. Doris's eyes flashed differently than my mother's. She often wore red and years after she, Elsie, and my mother died, the other aunts told me that Doris had been a flirt.

Blond, blue-eyed Marjorie came next. Twice widowed and once divorced. Dressed sensibly and played, "All the Nice Girls Love a Sailor" on the organ before she turned one hundred.

Then it was my mother Ethel, with her alluring looks, soft voice, and prowess in both the domestic and artistic domains. She could never learn how to whistle or blow bubbles with bubble gum but she did learn how to ride a two-wheeler bike when I got my first one. We both had scabbed knees.

Mother could sew anything and seldom used a pattern. She knit, embroidered, crocheted, hooked, and quilted, though failed in her attempts to have her only child recognize the fun in creating original works of art like her own. My mother had a soft voice, beautifully shaped hands and nails and a soft touch when tying my scarf, or turning me around after I'd tried on a half-finished dress she was making for me.

Two younger enchantress sisters were blond Dora, fair-skinned, blue-eyed, intelligent and the elegant brunette, dark-skinned Brownie, who I can still see playing "Nola" on the piano. They both lived to their mid-nineties.

My mother had color sense. Perhaps it was from mixing watercolors or the smelly oil paints she sometimes used. But I think it was from her love of flowers, which she'd grown up with. Her dad was an effective gardener. Though my grand-mother may have plotted the shape of the beds and type of flowers grown, he was the man to get the results. I sniffed his early tomato plants in his garden greenhouse and played in his waving asparagus beds. I was a pre-teen when my grandparents died so this guess for my mother's unusual color sense could be faulty.

I wish I had realized when I was young, how very special she was.

Don't cry because it's over; smile because it happened. — Anonymous

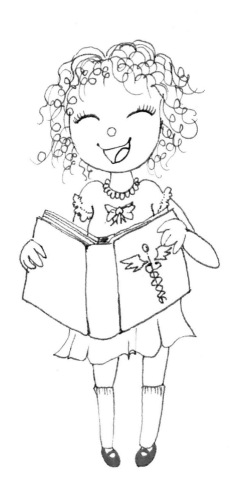

Grandpa Farrell's at Christmas

I was six, that nineteen thirty-four Christmas at Grandpa Farrell's, my father's childhood home at the top of Griersen Hill in Edmonton.

Seven of Grandpa's nine children had gathered with their families. There would have been ten adults and nine children. I was one of the younger ones.

After the complete turkey dinner at noon, we all trooped from the coal-scented dining room with its fireplace keeping only one end of the room warm, to the frigid parlor. You could almost see your breath and Aunt Lillian wrapped an extra shawl around squirming cousin Robert George. The room was formal, with stiff maroon velvet chairs, horsehair-stuffed love-seats protected by antimacassars, and an upright piano with oversized sheet music rumpling along its ledge.

All my uncles, except one, smoked, and ashtrays overflowed as the grandchildren performed an impromptu concert.

Uncle Russell had four children, the most in our family. His eldest was, we were all told, a child prodigy. Russell was a traveling salesman. Not the kind who sullies farmers' daughters, but one who was also known in the family as the mad scientist. One of his products was embalming fluid. It was said he had a bad batch one time, which tended to turn the dear departed yellow, so he turned this to his advantage and sold it as a special product to the Chinese market in Vancouver. He also made a product that cleaned the inside of oil tanks at refineries. As far as I know, they were different formulas.

Uncle Russell's daughter Eileen, the prodigy, performed first on the piano, rocking back and forth over the ivories, elbows splayed, head cocked as though listening for whispering piano beetles. She played the "Moonlight Sonata" by ear and I forget which, but an older male cousin recited the "Cremation of Sam McGee" from beginning to end.

When my turn came, I had prepared no memory work and had yet to start piano lessons.. I don't know what my mother thought I would come up with. Undaunted, I decided to show off my new reading skills. I hefted the heavy red *Home Medical* book, opened it at random and proceeded to read, carefully sounding out the words phonetically, as I'd been recently taught. My uncles, who'd been dozing, came to life. Uncle Russell's bald pate shone, his round face got red and he whacked my dad on the arm; my cousins, who were old enough, tittered; my mother said, "Thank you dear. Very good. That's enough." And I got the biggest round of applause of the day for my carefully enunciated elocution on the male reproductive system.

> *Reading is to the mind what exercise is to the*
> *body*. — Sir Richard Steele, Tatler, 1710

Mushroom Sundays

None of our Sundays were the same, but some favorite summer Sunday mornings were when my daddy and I would drive out to a farmer's cow pasture somewhere just south and east of what's now the city of St. Albert.

He held apart the barbed-wires on the fence, with a foot down and a hand up, while I held the skirt of my sky-blue Shirley Temple dress close to me to keep it from tearing as I crawled through the hole. Then it was, "Heads down, watch for mushrooms and cow pies." He secretly watched for the resident bull. We hunted the musky mushrooms in the lumpy field then placed them carefully in brown paper bags. These edible fungi were a favorite food of my dad's and he was very particular about only saving the freshest, bug-free, pink-gilled specimens.

The most exciting-looking mushrooms, though almost gross, were the giant puffballs, which we occasionally picked. I think my dad must have felt the same as I, a mouthful was just too much, and my mother didn't know enough in those days, to slice, egg-batter, crumb, and fry them.

When we returned with our bags full, Mummy would melt knobs of butter in the black iron frying pan. After cleaning the mushrooms with a damp cloth, she'd slice them into the frothing butter, all the while stirring and telling us, "I can't *stand* the smell *or* taste of these things," and my daddy and I would be waiting, waiting, while our little house was permeated with the essence of wild mushroom perfume. Then we salted and white-peppered the slithery slices and were a club of two.

Seeing is deceiving. It's eating that's believing. —James
Thurber, *Further Fables for Our Time*, 1956

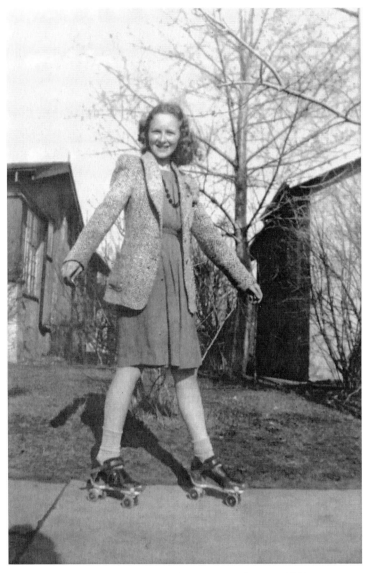

Joyce roller skates across from field — Garneau 1938

Raspberries

Raspberries turned my father, an otherwise saintly man, into a subversive thief. His favorite dessert was fresh raspberries on vanilla ice cream. I can see him grinning, sitting at the breakfast nook, his white shirt sleeves rolled up, shirt unbuttoned so I could glimpse a bit of blond chest hair, the hair on his head graying and cut so short as to be almost invisible. His light blue eyes crinkled, and he said to my mother "We have quite the crop this year."

I was silent one day when I saw him leaning into the straggly raspberry patch along the length of our garage. From my supine position on the green and white striped canvas swing I saw the bowl beside his feet was empty. He seemed to be on his own private feeding frenzy, only picking berries for immediate consumption. Presently, apparently temporarily satisfied, I saw him stroll into the lane where he stalled in front of our own spreading raspberry canes ,which had crammed their way through our tall cream painted fence. Then I saw his head drift slowly east, past the next-door neighbor's spreading fruit and I wondered if Mrs. McCauley could see him from her kitchen window. Then his head re-appeared. He paused at our property, our gate clicked open and shut and he carried a full bowl of perfect specimens to the kitchen as an offering to my mother who also had a fondness for his favorite fruit.

Slut Red Raspberries in Chardonnay Jelly
(from "Forever Summer" by Nigella Lawson, 2002)

Serves 6
- 1 bottle good Chardonnay wine
- 1 ½ c. raspberries
- 1 vanilla pod, split lengthwise
- 3 gelatin leaves
- 9 oz. berry sugar
- cereal or whipping cream to serve

1. Steep wine and berries in bowl for ½ hour. Strain wine into saucepan. Put raspberries to one side. Heat wine with vanilla pod. Steep off heat for 15 minutes

2. Soak gelatin leaves in cold water 5 minutes.

3. After removing vanilla pod from wine, reheat and stir in sugar. Boil only if you want to lose the alcohol. Add 1/3 of hot wine to wrung-out gelatin leaves in a pitcher and stir to dissolve, then add this mixture back into the rest of the wine and stir well.

(I love this squishing of the gelatin leaves. Not sure what it reminds me of. It's as though I'm doing something forbidden and I'm getting away with it.)

4. Strain into large jug.

5. Place raspberries equally, into 6 clear glass serving bowls and pour strained wine over the top.

6. Set in fridge at least 3 hours or a day ahead. Take out of fridge 15 minutes before serving.

7. Serve with cream in a jug and let people pour this into the fruit-jeweled jelly as they eat.

Raspberry Cream Brule (thanks to Judy Schultz)

Serves 2

- 2 c. ripe raspberries
- ½ c sour cream or yogurt
- 2 tsp. white sugar
- 1 tsp. vanilla
- 2 tsp. brown sugar

1. Put berries in 3 heat-proof dishes

2. Sweeten sour cream or yogurt with white sugar and stir in vanilla.

3. Put in dishes on top of berries.

4. Sprinkle brown sugar and broil till melted.

5. Serve immediately or just sprinkle on brown sugar at last minute and don't broil.

> *Part of the secret to success in life is to eat what you like and let the food fight it out inside.* — Mark Twain 1835-1910

If your life is burning well, poetry is just the ash. — Leonard Cohen

But Once Upon a Time

she never had to worry about
where the rent money was coming from
or the tedium of turnips cabbage potatoes
or baloney the only meat
overnight it seemed
but unknown to old friends
she stood in line at food banks wearing her
front edge frayed thirty-five year old Holt Renfrew coat
bought after late husband's salary raise
she had no teacher nurse stenographer tickets for jobs
besides too old but not old enough
not quite a senior
straight grey hair now trimmed with nail scissors
used to have weekly root tint manicure pedicure
trips to belize umbria and broadway
former home renovated with polished granite counters
air conditioning and cleaning ladies
now an apartment over a pizza pick-up
stair treads dipped and dirty
she works as a kitchen aid
in an old folks' home
her only child volunteers for rape victims
in congo
she emails from library computer
tells him how life continues
to tick along nicely
with news of old neighbors and
child's friends

The Cocktail Apron

It was useless. Pale pink, see-through organza. Full-blown roses with fresh green leaves and prickled stems covered the surface of this excuse for an apron. She had hand-painted it. Oils I think. No bib. After all, it wasn't intended as a slurp-catcher which she needed years later in her last days in a hospital. When a hand wiped over the apron, it slid, showing grease wouldn't adhere as it could on my mother's everyday aprons. These were embroidered, some, like her bleached flour-sack tea towels, with kittens performing the rigid tasks of the week above the hand-stitched days of the week. *Monday, washing. Tuesday, ironing. Wednesday, cleaning. Thursday, baking. Friday, shopping. Saturday, sewing /gardening. Sunday, church/rest*, which was not quite accurate, but it would have been too much to fit in "*visiting &/or big dinner for extended family.*"

My mother was glamorous. I once heard someone say, "*Ethel is so beautiful. The child looks just like the father.*" She had black wavy hair, a long neck, big brown eyes, wide smile, beautiful hands and a flapper figure. But she didn't act like a flapper, or what I imagine flappers to have been like from watching the best of *Masterpiece Theatre* plays of that era. This seems the most accurate view I'll ever have, although I was in this world in the late twenties and thirties. I now think, even though I was an only child and am told they are observant, that I was oblivious of much that went on around me.

But that cocktail apron. Scrumptiously beautiful. She wore it when they entertained. Fastened in the back with a wide bow. When I see it in my mind's eye, it's as though it was a pale pink butterfly fluttering gently from side to side. I can imagine a man's eyes glued to that bow until she turned her head, glanced over her shoulder at him, raised her beautifully arched eyebrows and said, "More tea? . . . Pie?"

She was known for her fine baking — angel food cakes and pies. And no Mixmasters in those days. She even made these cakes and pies to order for a friend's husband whose wife had other interests than baking. Not, I want you to know, that there was anything *ever* in these acts of kindness which could be gossiped about. I know this for a fact. I've talked to their daughters about the pie occasions and we all agree, shake our heads up and down, "Yes, purely platonic."

My blond, blue-eyed dad adored her. A cousin told me just the other day "Everyone knew your parents' marriage was a great love affair." When I asked, she then proceeded to tell me which of my aunts' and uncles' marriages on Dad's side were rocky.

Did Dad get excited when she tied on that see-through cocktail apron? I've heard that women wanting to rejuvenate their marriages have been advised to greet their tired homecoming husbands at the door stark naked except for an apron. Mother's rose-strewn butterfly bowed cocktail apron could fit that occasion, but I am *ashamed* of myself that I would even *think* of such a thing.

> *"If a woman hasn't got a tiny streak of a harlot in her, she's a dry stick as a rule."*
> — D.H.Lawrence, *Pornography and Obscenity*

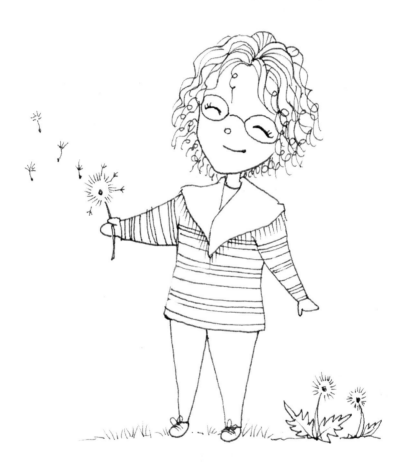

Dandelions

an egg cup holds
short-stemmed
spring dandelions
picked by
tiny hands
from along the
warm garage wall
thrust up
sticky
sap stained
fingers
squeezed bright yellow
the mother holds
these shaggy gifts
under her child's chin
says
you like butter
don't you
the child laughs
years later
tests her own child's chin

Fiction

That's the Way it Is —
Hi Gum Yeung

I thought we'd got away with it, but had known deep down that we couldn't keep it a secret forever. Much as we'd tried. But who would have thought? I finished wiping the granite counter-tops in our newly renovated kitchen. Our super-quiet German dishwasher was doing its super-quiet thing.

I looked over at Robert stretched out in his leather chair, his white-socked feet propped on an old camel saddle. I'd given our daughter Brenda her dinner-on-the-run earlier since she had to go back to university for an evening lab. Then we ate, and right after, our son Michael burst in with his bombshell. He began talking on his way to the fridge, his normal route, then took out a Tupperware jug of orange juice and lifted it to his lips. I thought, "Why don't girls ever do this?" His Adam's apple bobbed while he glugged, briefly stopping his chatter. Then he began again, grinning and shaking his head in disbelief at what he had seen and heard that afternoon at the university book store. I got a tight feeling in my throat and knew tears might start coming but I gulped and said, "Most peculiar — maybe there is a connection somewhere." Robert was quiet, just, "Really, Michael?" but I saw him pale and I could only think what he must be thinking.

*   *   *

I flicked back to our late seventies perfect high school days when I had said to Robert, "You are Lion," and he had said, "You are Panther." Romantically appropriate endearments, we'd thought. He with that thick red-blond mane and side-burned cheeks, as many cheeks were in those late seventies days. I had my same black hair in bangs and Oriental eyes. We were "the couple" in high school. I adored him in the Mackenzie tartan kilt he wore at weekend parades and I became used to the skirl of bagpipe music though I preferred Joan Baez, Joni Mitchell and the Beatles. His Scottish background showed in his solid body, and in his self-assured manner. He was the newly elected student union president and the tallest guy on the basketball team. I was the yearbook director and did well at track. My specialty was the hundred-yard dash.

We met in halls, held hands, talked on the phone and studied together when we could. No cellphones in those days. Everyone knew it was true love. We had been told that grade ten and eleven girls sighed, "Robert and Kim, Robert and Kim," and dreamed they too could have a romance such as ours.

*   *   *

I remember clearly, it was the beginning of March, before spring exams. The windows in the study hall were frosted lightly at their bottoms and the school's yard lights had just turned off. They'd been shining on heavy snow from an early spring blizzard. Robert and I had a free period first thing and we always met here to whisper and write notes. This day Robert rushed up to me, clearly upset. "Well Kim, I've done it, the news is out. To my family, anyway."

"Robert, what happened?"

"Well, we had Mom's usual big Sunday dinner and I'd been waiting for the right moment to tell, you know, we've talked of the best way for days now, when Mom said, 'Robert, are you coming down with something? You haven't finished your flapper pie, your favorite dessert. What's the trouble dear?' Uh, gulp. I looked at the three of them, Mom, Dad and Mary, sitting there like they didn't have a worry in the world and how they'd be so — Idonno — sad, mad, so I just blurted. 'You must know, Kim and I love each other very much. She's pregnant and we want to get married and keep the baby.'"

"Oh Robert — hi gum yeung — that's the way it is."

"Before I finished, Dad had pushed back his chair and leaned over at me. His face redder and redder, like it does Kim, and he shouted, 'You what? You think it's that simple?' and then he got white and he plunked down in his chair. Kim, I thought maybe he was having a heart attack. Then I thought maybe he'd cry. I've never seen him cry. But he didn't, he just got quiet. 'You're both only seventeen and a half. Robert, you've got a wonderful future ahead of you. There's no way you're going to have a . . .'" Robert's face flushed.

"And what? What else did he say?"

I remember, he looked down at his feet, "Sorry Kim . . . 'a Chink wife and a half-cast bastard to hold you back.' Mom was saying, 'Sshh, Sshh Hamish,' and Mary was crying and it was awful. They're going to talk to your parents."

"Robert, it'll be awful. When?"

"Tomorrow, I think."

"Well, tell them I haven't broken the news yet to Mother and Pa. Surely your dad'll wait for a day. I'll go straight home after school. We're eating early tonight and I'll tell them. Wonder if it'll be the same with them." The bell rang. We clasped hands, and kissed the air toward each other. "Don't forget — don't let them phone 'til tomorrow." And we went our separate ways.

I thought about my parents, Sam and Lily Wong. The path they'd taken in life. They'd each immigrated from southern China with their families landing somehow in Edmonton and after marriage both had numerous jobs until they became managers at the Chinese Benevolent Society's Elder's residence in Chinatown. When I started high school, they changed direction to run a herbal shop where not only the Chinese community listened to what Pa said, but also Occidentals who were beginning to believe in acupuncture felt it was the next step for them to look at his herbal remedies. As an only child I grew up with the large community of "aunts" and "uncles" in the residence. I'd seen what happened when a befuddled elder dropped her slipper in the toilet and the overflow ran down the hall and the stairs and I had to help my mother and father deal with the result. I saw when Uncle Ling died, toppling down the stairs, his frail old bones breaking like a tiny chicken's. I saved old Aunt Em, toothless and grinning, after she'd wandered out the front door onto the street miraculously evading squealing cars on her way to her long lost market garden of forty years ago.

I sat with my parents in the kitchen of our apartment over the store. It smelled of the ten-spice mixture I made up for my mother every week. Robert had told me once, "I love your smell Kim — I can tell it's you when you come up behind me." I wondered if that was a good thing. When I first started at the big high school I didn't like it when my mother insisted on including those tiny dumplings in my packed lunches, and I didn't like it when I couldn't always get to Robert's special Saturday parades because I was working in the store. I hated the arguments about my choice of clothes, especially the new Carnaby Street mini-skirts, although I'd read this wasn't just a cultural clash. I hated my poker-straight black hair when I couldn't back-comb it into black froth. It would only twang out and look silly.

I'd put off this quiet confession to my parents for too long. I knew how deeply disappointed they'd be. Since Robert's parents knew and were going to summon my family for a show-down, they must be told.

"May I have more tea please mother?" I watched while Mother's small hands lifted the blue and white teapot. Fragrant green tea filled my tiny cup. The rice steamer's lid was jiggling while chopped bok choy, chicken livers, ginger root and bean sprouts waited to be cooked in the old wok. "Pa, Mother, I have something to tell that you won't want to hear. You must know Robert and I love each other very much. Well, we're going to have a baby and we want to get married. Robert's parents want to meet you and talk about it. They'll be phoning you prob-ably tomorrow."

Neither of them acted as though they had heard me. Looking at one another, they lifted their cups to their lips and took dainty sips. I knew I would always think of this day when in the future I drank tea with my parents. Still they did not speak. They were thinking, considering. It was Pa who finally spoke. I could tell he was moved. He was not the inscrutable man after all whom Robert had met only a few times.

"Ah, ah, my fragrant little flower." He'd called me this for as long as I could remember and I reveled in the idea of being like the roses my mother cultivated beside the lane in the tiny back yard along with lily-of-the-valley and bright pink petunias. His eyes were sparkling, though no tears fell. "We should have guessed this could happen. We should have kept you apart. In Canada, you're too young to marry." And he lowered his head, looking at the dregs in his teacup.

My mother stopped drinking tea and sat, still as a tiny Buddha. All she said was, "Ah, ah, Kim, I'm thinking." While I knew she was every bit as upset as Pa, like women through the ages, I imagined she was thinking practically and said, "I'll ask Min. No close relatives to take the baby — Min can't. But Kim you could stay with her in Vancouver or Min can find a home for you 'til it's over and the child can be put up for adoption. Half-a-loaf," she muttered and, "hard to place."

"Half-a-loaf, half-a-loaf" echoed through my head. "Hard to place." I knew three things for sure. I wouldn't have an abortion. If we couldn't keep the baby, I'd see it got a good home and I knew I wouldn't let this destroy us. My Lion and I would always be together.

*   *   *

The showdown began: "How do you do Sam," Hamish Mackenzie said, shaking hands, "and Lily." When he grasped my mother's hand I noticed her slight wince. He must have a squeezed too tightly. But that was his way — Hamish was too hearty. Robert told me he'd been in a Scottish regiment in the Canadian army during World War Two, probably as a blustering but brave Colonel. He lived through the European conflict with a small shrapnel wound on his left wrist, and returned to Canada where he was employed at a German steel-pipe plant, as their overseas sales manager. He'd done all right. Married cushiony Agnes, who knew how to run a household and was a good mother to Robert and their daughter Mary.

Their home was on a curving street overlooking the silted North Saskatchewan river. In the living room tall wrought iron lamps with fringed shades cast yellow light on the Danish modern furniture so popular then. I could tell mother was thinking, "Bad feng shui."

I watched my parents, so tiny on the modern sofa, their backs touching the grey wool fabric. Their feet, especially Mother's, hanging in mid-air. Then they had to hunker forward, planting their feet firmly on the layered blue and red Persian carpets scattered over the highly polished floors.

Mr. McKenzie looked at my parents. He was probably thinking, "Pretty nervous. They'll agree with us. They won't want a mixed-race grandchild either."

Mrs. McKenzie announced, "I'll just get the coffee."

Holding hands, Robert and I took our places on a black striped loveseat. Darling Robert held his head high, long legs thrust out in front of him. He drew them back when his mother reappeared bearing a large black tole tray loaded with a pewter coffee pot, cream and sugar, pink and white Messien cups and saucers and a platter of biscuits. She placed these on the small Danish table and sat leaning forward. Robert's sister Mary wasn't around, though I supposed she was hovering within earshot, taking in every word. She was a good kid. Robert was quite confident that she wouldn't tell even her best friend about tonight.

"Lily, do you take cream and sugar?"

"Yes, thanks."

Untangling his long length, Robert arose and served the tea and passed cookies to everyone. His parents locked eyes and his father began: "Now folks, we've got a pretty serious problem here. As I see it, there's only one solution. No plan to terminate the pregnancy — an abortion? That's so isn't it Kim?"

I remember feeling hot and knew I was blushing. I whispered, "No, Mr. McKenzie. Not that."

"Okay, Sam do you have somewhere she can go to have the baby and then put it up for adoption? These two are far too young to consider marriage and keeping the kid. You must agree?"

Softly, but firmly, Pa said, "Well, Mr. McKenzie, of course Lily and I have talked it over and we haven't phoned her yet, but we think Kim can go to her Aunt Min in Vancouver. She'll arrange a good home for her 'til it's over. We are honorable people. Hate lies. But we feel somehow we have to make up a story for

Kim that's believable. This pregnancy must be kept a secret. We want your family to promise you will go along with it for her sake as well as for your son's."

Robert squeezed my hand, and I remember being both surprised and dismayed. I'd heard my parents talking quietly in their bedroom the night before, though they hadn't said anything to me at breakfast that morning or in the silent car on our way to this meeting. I thought somehow Pa and Mother might come up with a plan that would be the best for all. This made it definite. There was absolutely no possibility we could marry and keep the baby. If Pa said it, it was so. I vowed I wouldn't cry since this would make it harder for Robert, but tears began sliding down my cheeks. I let them. I didn't want to make a show of wiping them away so they slipped off my chin into the cold coffee cup I held in front of my tender breasts.

"Sam — glad you agree. Yes, Agnes and I want the whole thing hush-hushed as much or more than you do," and glaring at the two young people, he pointed and waggled his finger, "And you two, carry on as usual at school, so no one will think anything's wrong, and I mean it. It's now adult business and we'll tell you what's going to happen when we know. Do you agree Robert? Kim? Sam? Lily?"

Pa shook his head, up and down, then from side to side. "Ah, ah, it's the only way. The families must keep this in our own walls. As you say, these two have long lives ahead of them. When we make the arrangements, I'll let you know." And he stood up, my mother at his side.

Mother came over to us and quietly said, "I'm sad for you, Robert, but maybe some day there will be a happy ending." I was dumbfounded but grateful to my mother for recognizing Robert's role in this drama. Blinking goodbye, our subdued little family retrieved our coats and boots and departed into the slushy night.

*   *   *

The story was to be thus: A friend of my Aunt Min in Vancouver had a difficult pregnancy. She badly needed help with ten and eight year-old girls 'til the baby arrived and then for a couple of months afterwards, through August. I would be the mother's helper. The money I got for this would help towards my first year of university. I was to finish the school year by correspondence courses, then apply to go to the University of Alberta in the fall.

On my last night at home, both Mother and Pa made a noble effort to be cheerful. Pa had closed the store early and Mother had made one of my favorite dinners — hoisin pork with tree ears, though I had trouble choking it down. "Kim," Pa said, "It's for less than five months. You'll see, the time will go quickly — you'll be busy and useful." He smiled, "That Min, she does know how to arrange things." At bedtime my mother watched me standing sideways in front of the bathroom mirror checking my stomach's progress, and said "Ah, ah, Kim, you're strong, strong enough to bear what's ahead. I'm thinking of the end of your time in Vancouver. Keep thinking '*hi gum yeung*.' That's the way it is, *hi gum yeung*," and she put her arms around me, kissing me, something she hadn't done since I was a young child. I lay awake in my narrow bed, too distraught to fall asleep. I left the window blind up to let the yard light beam into my room, across the bulletin board nailed to the wall over my desk. I stared at its notices of pep rallies, track and field ribbons and medallions and one faded carnation and heather corsage from a Scottish Society 'do.' I wouldn't be going to our grad party.

There were spaces where I'd removed pictures. These were carefully stuck in the small tartan album Robert had given me, which was now in my suitcase. There was a picture of Robert in mid-air, his long arm arcing a basketball into the hoop; one of him grinning at me while he whacked his big drum, his kilt flipping to one side while he paraded on Robbie Burns Day. There was a picture of us together, Robert behind me, his arms wrapping me with his love, both of us laughing at the camera. One of me and my parents standing proudly opening day, in front of our store under the expensive green awning. I was thirteen. Little did I know what lay ahead, though for whom does that matter? And finally, a picture of me with my friend Jennie on our first day of high school. My father had surprised us at the bus stop and clicked the camera just as I was about to take the first step up into the bus. Jennie was right behind me. We both looked surprised. I remember feeling so nervous and excited. I met Robert that day. We were in registration lines next to each other and got talking. I liked him right from the start.

*   *   *

Less than a week later, Aunt Min had found a place for me and Robert picked me up at six in the morning, an hour and a half before the Greyhound bus was to leave. Hard to believe we wouldn't see or hold one another for nearly five months. Hard to say, "*Hi gum yeung*," so we ended up with, "I'll love you forever."

"I'll love you forever," and it was time for me to board the bus A long trip. I'd only suffered mild morning sickness in my first two months and now though my breasts were sore and my stomach starting to thicken, I felt alive and well. I wondered how this could be. I made up my mind that for the next five months, besides my schoolwork and duties with my employer's family, I would think and do whatever I could in order to have a perfect child. I would eat only nutritious food, exercise and get enough sleep. I would talk to this baby, telling his or her the story of its parents great love for one another. Besides doing my schoolwork, I would play great music and read only great literature. I would watch sunsets and never get angry. This baby would have both our genes and I would make sure that our precious love child would always be nourished without negative thoughts. I would not allow it. I would not.

Aunt Min met me at the Vancouver bus depot. I hadn't seen her since I was little. Though her hair was grey, she looked like mother. Their voices were similar but my mother's accent was more pronounced. Mother had told me it was her sister Min who'd arranged the introduction of my parents twenty years ago. She said that she and Min had been at a Sunday dim sum in Edmonton, and Min had said ,"I think you two should meet, " and then she left them alone. Look what happened: a solid loving marriage. And now she was managing my life too. I hoped the results would be as good.

"You're staying with me, Kim, for the next two nights so I'll have a chance to show you a bit of Vancouver. We're within walking distance of the O'Briens where you're going to live. We'll go and meet them tomorrow afternoon and you'll move in on Sunday."

When we walked up the path to the big grey and white house, we heard a dog's deep bark. Strange to think I would be living in this big house and I'd be in charge of two children, shopping for groceries and cooking meals. Mrs. O'Brien, or rather, Dr. O'Brien, met us at the door. She wore faded denim maternity overalls and was wrestling with a big golden Labrador dog who wasn't very well trained, I thought. "Stay, Rory, stay," and she held his collar until he finally sat on his haunches, panting and looking at us with a mixture of pleasure and suspicion. "Come in, come in. He sometimes escapes, and it's such a nuisance to have to go after him." Once the door had closed behind us, the dog had separate sniffs, wagged his tail and trotted off around a corner ahead of us, his claws clicking on the tile floor. He evidently knew where we were to go. Dr. O'Brien had us follow her into the kitchen-family room.

Even with the grey overcast sky through the skylights, I felt the warmth of the room. We sat and had tea and some broken store-bought cookies. Dr. O'Brien laughed and said she hoped her supplies would be in better shape once I got my act together. That's how I would come to think of this period in my life: as a play, with acts and scenes. Like act two, scene two. There would be more acts and scenes in this play, but act three would be when I returned home to Robert and we would have scenes including our own future family and then at the curtain's end, we would be old people together holding hands bowing in front of a red curtain and that would be that.

"Pardon?" I said, "No, no thanks, no more tea." Dr. O'Brien and Aunt Min had been talking and I had tuned out, though I don't think for long. I hoped I hadn't missed anything crucial.

Rory barked and Dr. O'Brien said, "That'll be the kids. Their Dad went to pick them up from their diving lessons. Kim, Min says you can, so you'll be expected to do some of the driving. We'll figure out the car situation and your B.C. license by next week. Here they are. Maureen, Sheila, meet Kim. She's going to live with us and help Mummy out. Kim this is my husband, Donald."

I said hello and smiled at each of the children, then rose to shake hands with the man of the house. Although I had been worried about this new life I was to be briefly dropped into, I felt happy with my first encounter with the family. It was explained that Dr. O'Brien was going to continue with her medical practice at least part time, while she could. She'd need to rest when she was home. Mr. O'Brien said "Hi Min, thanks for bringing her. Kim, since I'm an architect, my schedule can be erratic sometimes too. Like today, I had to get a neighbor to drop the kids off, and then I picked them up. Darling," he said to his wife, "we stopped for pizza on the way home. Didn't think you'd have dinner waiting."

"Good guess, dear. Kim, I don't much like cooking and meals. Actually, I hate it, so you're it. Okay? I'll make a list of the things we like and don't like. Don will tell you how we handle the house money. C'mon kids, let's show Kim her room."

We twisted down some iron stairs to the basement and my room, complete with bed, dresser, TV and desk. Mr. O'Brien was at the end of the line. "That's one of mine," he said, pointing to a bright yellow and blue canvas that nearly covered the wall above my desk.

Looking at the painting, his wife said, "Don's really an artist working as an architect. Isn't it great? We thought you should have something cheerful since we know you're used to Alberta's blue skies, so we all chose this." Their Dad grinned. Dr. O'Brien put an arm around each of the girl's shoulders and said, "They helped me pick out the lamp and the new duvet cover and the towels too in your bathroom. I hope you like pink, Kim."

"Thanks, I love it and what a good lamp. You know I'll be doing a lot of homework at night-time when you're sound asleep." Maureen and Sheila smiled broadly and I knew we'd get along.

We went upstairs again, to the front hall. Dr. O'Brien said, "Thanks Min. I'm sure everything will work out for all of us — and Kim, you know I'm your doctor, don't you?"

It was better than I could have hoped for. I could pretty well make up my own daily routine, I felt well and she would be my doctor. I liked her from the beginning. Different from the brusque man I'd gone to back home. I had felt his displeasure when he examined me, and the way he said, "About three months," as though he was talking to a dumb promiscuous kid.

One day melted into another. As Dr. O'Brien's stomach expanded, so did mine. I'd bought duck-boots and was getting accustomed to Vancouver's drizzle. When the children went with their parents to visit grandparents on weekends, I usually walked the sea walk. I wasn't accustomed to that peculiar and, at first I thought, nasty smell. Gradually, though, as I gazed at the waves, became used to their incessant lapping, and watched the noisy gulls swooping, the sea air became bracing. It made me want to walk faster and think harder. To my surprise, I grew fond of the ocean.

Maureen and Sheila were good kids. I'd taught them some skipping games I played when I was little and we went to a park by the ocean across the Lion's Gate to fly kites. They often came to my room and I told them about Robert. They looked at my pictures of him, one on my night table, the other on my desk, and I told them about the pictures in my tartan album.

Some weeks before Dr. O'Brien's baby was due, she found out it was dead. She had to wait till she went into labor to deliver it. A boy. I tried to comfort the children when Mr. O'Brien told me. He had talked so often about the child his wife was carrying. He was more outwardly emotional than his wife. Not that Dr. O'Brien was cold, anything but, but she seemed to have better control of her emotions than he did. Maybe they teach that in medical school, but don't have to in architecture. You could hardly have doctors crying all over the place. Anyway, I felt most sorry for him though I knew how disappointed they all were and there I sat. A puffed balloon with stick arms and legs. Young, healthy, but carrying a child I couldn't keep. My baby was due in two months and I wondered if Dr. and Mr. O'Brien would want me lumping around, reminding them of their own baby every time they looked at me. But no, when she came home, thin but still smiling, she said "Of course you must stay. I need you. We all need you."

Tulips in the garden had finished blooming and were replaced by pink petunias, like at home, and white asters.

Blackberries were ripening along the path by the railroad tracks, big and heavy. Nothing like the summer clusters of powdery Saskatoon berries my mother and I picked each year and bottled. I had the O'Briens eating my stir-fries though I went easy on the ten-spice mixture. Often the days were warm and sunny. I paddled in the pool with the children, and in spite of my tummy, they taught me how to dive. They liked me and I had grown to love their funny ways. At ten, Maureen was not much taller than her younger sister Sheila. She was a dark-haired, quick moving, quick-to-anger, quick-to-laugh girl, while Sheila was blond, tending toward chubbiness and at eight had turned into a bookworm. I shot baskets with Maureen while Sheila sat on the grass beside the driveway, reading yet another chapter book. I read to them both, at night, when neither of their parents could and that was my favorite time. I imagined the day when Robert and I would have our real life and I would be reading to our children. "I know it's going to happen. I know it." I would say to myself. At the same time I would apologize and pat my stomach, "It's okay little one, I'll make sure you have a wonderful family." Of course I had talked to Dr. O'Brien about our baby's adoption and she had explained a private adoption was a fairly straightforward process. Although in those days, a mixed race child was less likely to be snapped up than a white blue-eyed blond. She told me she would be on the lookout.

I asked her if the way I was conducting myself, with my diet, exercise and especially my thoughts, would mean this baby could be special and she replied, "All babies are special Kim and I'm sure this one will thrive on his mother's special prenatal care." So that made me feel better, though she always made me feel better with her gentle touch when she examined me, and that smile and soft voice.

Mr. O'Brien tended to be a bit high-strung, but he was so energetic and he threw himself into his work and painting. When things were going well, he reminded me of Robert–that joy my Lion got from banging the drum and the look on his face after a good basketball game.

I had time in those days to think about such things — comparisons between people I loved and those I didn't know as well. It wasn't as though I was giving points, but just that I needed to gauge what I thought I wanted to be like, or our life together to be like. Maybe all women get this way when they're pregnant. I didn't know. I did know I wouldn't be pregnant again for at least three years. Depending on how things worked out for us at university. We'd marry the end of first year. I hoped *two can live as cheap as one* was true.

We wrote to each other every other day. On Sundays, we tried to reach each other without paper. Just by thoughts. Remember, this was in 1968, before instant communication.

Then on another examination day, Dr. O'Brien heard two heartbeats. She said it was a bit unusual to have found this out so late — in my eighth month. She'd been suspicious because of my size, though she figured my small body just carried differently. Would this mean the babies(!) would be more difficult to place in a good home?

I wrote to Robert and told him he was to be the father of twins in less than a month. I was getting pretty uncomfortable — puffing when I ran up the stairs from my room and the strings on my white cook's apron could barely tie in the back. I hadn't been able to see my feet for ages when I looked down and when I was laying in the bath the mound of babies above the water line made me giggle. The way it rose and subsided like the beginning of a stove-top chocolate pudding before it completely comes to a bubble. Robert should have been there to see. Those were busy little boys. More and more I told myself, "*Hi gum yeung*," and, "Think positive, think positive." It was harder, but somehow, if the babies got a good home, that was the best I could do for them. Time was close and so far Dr. O'Brien hadn't found the right family.

"We're going to take you in, Kim," was what she said.

"There's nothing wrong, is there Dr. O'Brien?"

"No, but it's time. I'll be there with you, Kim."

So there I was. It happened. After, it was a crystal-clear fog in my mind. I saw the babies, black hair plastered to their heads — I'd rather hoped they might have red hair. I'd tried to figure it out from a library book on genetics, and I knew it was most likely that straight black hair would dominate.

Dr. O'Brien sat on the edge of my bed in the private room she'd paid for and she took my hand. Mr. O'Brien stood beside her while Aunt Min sat expressionless on the chair beside the bed.

"Kim, we've talked to Min about it, but now we want to know your feelings. We know you're still in a euphoric state but we want your first reaction to...what do you think if Don and I adopt your boys? They'll be little brothers for Maureen and Sheila." I couldn't breathe. "You know what we're like, and we know you."

Don leaned over, "You know how I, we, have wanted a boy and to have two, well. We'll love them and raise them to be good people. Their father sounds like a great guy. Please Kim, say yes."

Dr. O'Brien squeezed my hand and said, "If it's both you and your family's wish to have this a lost portion of your lives, at least you'll know what kind of parents and home your sons will have. It should give you some peace of mind."

She was in tears and I was crying freely. All I could say was "I can't believe it." I looked at Aunt Min who was nodding her head up and down. But I said, "When must I say and when are you coming to see me again?"

"Soon — tomorrow."

"Would you, for Robert, for me, give the boys Scottish names? Would it be too odd for them to look Chinese, have Scottish first names with an Irish last name?"

*   *   *

The years flew. Starting with our first year; Robert got a hefty scholarship and I got a smaller one. Tuition was relatively cheap in 1979, so we managed. While we both ached at the thought of our sons, only I could picture quite clearly how Maureen and Sheila might be walking them back and forth in a twin baby carriage on the driveway or how Mr. O'Brien might have them in the car, waiting for the older children to come out of the rec center. I could see them sitting in the family room, early fall rain ticking on the skylight. Dr. O'Brien would be holding them and one at a time, giving them their bottles, kissing their fine black heads, while a stranger, my replacement, would be making a delicious dinner. The boys would be cooing and...I told myself, "Stop thinking this way. Stop it." Lucky Robert — he couldn't see what I could. When I left the O'Brien's we agreed we would not be in touch. This Act would be played in the dark.

*   *   *

In the spring of our first university year, we married. We got good summer jobs. Robert up north at an early oil sands plant which paid well and me as a lab assistant at the hospital which didn't pay as well but would look good on a resume. Another scene in Act Three. Robert teased me about my fantasy scripting of our life but I didn't stop. Sure the play had had some glitches but we were well on-track again. This time, we would have a planned baby. In our third year of university. And it came to pass. Michael, a beautiful black-haired baby with very large feet was born on the fifteenth of August 1973.

I thought of the two in Vancouver, but soon was able to dwell only on this baby. Somehow he sensed, I was sure, that he was a longed-for beloved child even before his birth. I followed the same prenatal dietary and mental rules, so knew I could do no more. Robert marveled at my pudding-bubbling stomach and he was in the birthing room with me.

Two years later, Brenda was born and was just as wanted and adored.

Everything was on track. We'd remodeled the little house by the university with a skylight like the O'Brien's. The children were healthy and doing well.

We both worked. Robert became a successful sanitary engineer, and traveled the north working with other environmentally-informed people. I had an interesting job as a counselor to unwed mothers. Nothing I'd started out doing, but somehow I found my correct niche. I was one of the few who often recommended to my girls that they think long and clearly about whether or not to keep their child. Of course, I never told this story. Times have changed, it seems either unwanted pregnancies produce war within families, the girl leaves home and they rarely reconcile, or parents are supportive or more often, young girls have abortions. In our day, parents had more say in their children's lives. Robert and I marvel at our parents' change of attitudes when we were married and produced legitimate grandchildren for them.

*   *   *

"This guy dropped his knapsack on my foot at the bookstore. Like looking in a mirror. He even said, 'there's another just like me at home in Vancouver. We must be *dopplegangers.*' Never heard that word before. Mom, they're three and a half years older than me. Their teeth have a space in the middle just like mine. Both of them. Bruce and Douglas. Incredible. We have to be related somehow. How many Chinese-Canadian guys six-foot plus do you see who look like me?"

It was time.

The next morning, at six o'clock, we woke Michael and Brenda.

"Your Dad and I have something we want to tell you..."

Love generously, praise loudly, live fully. — Elias Porter

That's Life

It was as good a day as any can be.

The young woman I was studies him as she has not studied him before. He is in the garage, its wide door open to a late October afternoon sun. Two little boys, one four the other two, paddle around him. The little one walks through a shaft of light beaming almost to the back of the space, noting his shadow, but too young to inquire about it. He is quiet. The older boy babbles. Question after question. "Daddy, why are you doing that? What's that thing? What will it do?"

I sit on the yellow brick back steps watching and listening. The baby, a fourteen-month-old girl, is due to wake from a too-late afternoon nap. She will probably be impossible at bedtime. I watch the man, my husband, and think: *How did I know? I didn't. I couldn't. That he would be such a good father.*

I never knew Hu's father, so didn't see what he learned at his own father's knee. I never knew the kind of patience he would show with our own young children. The clearness with which he explained, "Tommy, I'm oiling right in here — see — I squeeze a bit and tip and the drops go in this little hole so when Brucie pedals your old tricycle it will be easier for him. I think maybe we've left it out in the rain too often and that's not good for it, so we have to give it a drink of oil to make these parts here turn better. Brucie, climb up little guy, you're getting so big you can reach the pedals now. You couldn't do that a while ago — good going — can you pedal down the driveway?

I'll follow you so you don't land in the street. Okay partner, you follow us on your big trike."

The young woman I was smiles, looks down at my stained apron and thinks with satisfaction: *For once all is calm, dinner's in the oven, a roasting chicken, small potatoes, carrots and onions cooking in the same casserole. They'll all like it, except the onions.*

The young woman I was doesn't think about these two young boys growing up to ride large two-wheelers or, god forbid, motorcycles. She doesn't think of them behind the wheel of the family car, or with girlfriends. She certainly doesn't think that they might give us grandchildren. I think no further ahead than for picky details of new snowsuit for Tommy and the serviceable brown hand-me-down for Brucie. Jody will of course wear the rather boyish red suit a third time 'round, but she can wear a hand-knit bonnet of blue and white with embroidered pink daisies which has stretched from her infancy until now.

The young woman I was doesn't think about what trails we might travel and there is never a thought of losing a child, our own health, or when our parents will no longer be in our lives.

The young woman I was is not thinking of the big picture, only details, details, details.

*   *   *

Now, the old woman I am smiles when I think about that autumn day in nineteen fifty-three. It would have been close to Halloween and I could not know what would happen after trick-or-treating in the spooky dark, when Tommy and Brucie trundled down our street with their daddy. They were wearing clown costumes my mother made out of old sheets and calico scraps.

Next morning I found our two little boys in baby Jody's crib, where the trio were trading licks of suckers.

Later that day, Tommy was lethargic and when he bent his head forward, cried out in pain. All parents had been warned about this cruel symptom. Our pediatrician neighbor came to the house and pronounced, "It's polio." The fierce epidemic had struck our house. Our thoughts: *Tommy — Oh No. And what about Brucie and Jody?* We nursed Tommy at home for six days and five nights. On the sixth evening we took him to the Royal Alexandra hospital's quarantine entrance where we had to leave him. Poor little boy. He was whisked to an operating room.

In the middle of the night our exhausted pediatrician came to the door with, "We lost him."

A big picture detail.

> **I am not young enough to know every-**
> **thing.** — Oscar Wilde 1854-1900

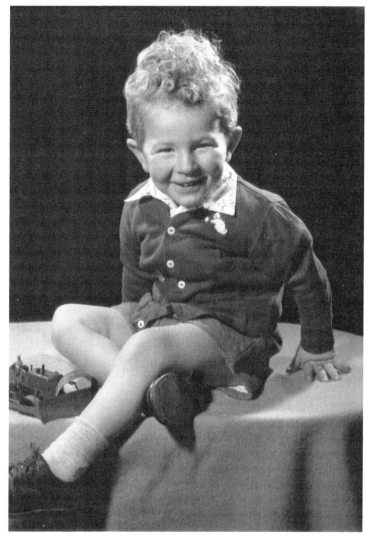

Tommy — 1952

A Pile of Pancakes

A pancake by any other name would smell as sweet. And they do. Flapjacks from the United States, crepes from France, tortillas from Mexico and blini from Russia.

Can you remember the smell of pancakes, bacon and coffee some Sunday mornings when you were very young? Your mother would sometimes dot the batter in the shape of a teddy bear, and you would watch the tiny bubbles appear on the moist surface. She would flip the whole critter over, his backside now rimmed and speckled with brown, and you would always eat more than she thought you could? Just like that little boy with the now politically incorrect name, wearing his red jacket, blue pants and purple shoes with crimson soles and crimson linings. Remember — after the tigers had melted into butter and his mother made pancakes and he ate one hundred and sixty-nine he was so hungry?

Can you imagine flapjacks cooked over an open fire on a dark morning in central British Columbia where leather-chapped grizzled cowboys wait hungrily, their stubbled faces deep-lined and tired from long days in the saddle at round-up-time?

Can you picture yourself in a small, mirrored bistro in Paris? Only locals know of it, though it's quite close to the Luxembourg Gardens. Your so-perfect waiter places two thin crepes before you with a flourish. They hold thin pencils of bright green asparagus and a sauce of such subtlety it cannot be described.

Can you imagine leaving your cold northern home for the Saturday morning Oaxaca market in southern Mexico? You're at one of the breakfast counters and you choose a dark brown ceramic bowl of foamy hot chocolate. With it you have a tortilla, small and crisp, drizzled with black bean puree and green salsa topped with chunks of a mild white cheese.

Can you feel yourself in New York, not Russia, but in a Russian restaurant? You're about to be served a tiny leavened pancake called blini. Your red-rimmed, warm plate arrives with a circle of pale gold blini. In the center of this circle is a pile of thin, rosy-peach smoked salmon slices looking like a tiny doll's rumpled silk scarf.

I tell you...a pancake by any other name...

To know how to order and enjoy good food is part of a civilized education.

— Lady Blanche Hozier (mother of Clementine Churchill)

The Thumb Thimble

a thumb thimble
with a Welsh symbol
could have been for stitching
lamb leather
into breeches
for her man
fighting the English
and she wiped her eyes
as she sewed
mad that it was
necessary
and she sewed a wish
into the right hand
corner of the garment
to keep him safe
she hasn't told him
he's to be a father
it will be their first
kicks early
hopes it will be a girl who will not
go to war
who can put this thimble on her thumb
push the needle
make the magic
wishes but

it's too soon to worry
about a son-in-law

*One merit of poetry few persons will deny: it says more
and in fewer words than prose.* —Voltaire

Hidden Bar Ranch*

Chapter 1

What matters are the memories. All we are left with. For those days between 1954 and 1981, the days of the Hidden Bar Ranch, life created its own whirling momentum that left so many memories.

Now, so many years later, I can see how I was caught up in my husband's dreams. I had no unusual ones of my own. I'd dreamed of a loving husband and healthy children. The dreams I married were as contagious as chicken pox though only sometimes as irritating.

From snippets of our life at Hidden Bar, I can now see what was happening. But did I relish those times as much as I could? Did I know what I was living? Did I know — truly know — those times would be a large part of the "stuff of life?" Did I know how I would fare as the wife of a dreamer always onto a new idea? And ideas for things I knew nothing of?

These are my memories and they are rich and good, though when I zero-in, they aren't without the tension of wondering.

In the beginning, our headquarters consisted of an original settler's cabin, walls chinked with mud, then whitewashed as it awaited new occupants. No indoor plumbing or electricity. Sagging, paint-deprived outbuildings and cattle pens wanting attention. Before long, we would meet male neighbors who came to see who had bought Chris's farmstead.

Hidden Bar Ranch the biggest story of the three. The three ranches: Hidden Bar Ranch east of Edmonton, Stampede Cattle Station south of Calgary, and Paradise Ranch in south-central British Columbia. It was the first. In 1954 we scraped up all we could afford for a few acres of gray, wooded land east of Edmonton. At the end, Hidden Bar had three thousand acres and everything that went with it — machinery, cattle, horses, barns, wells, bunk-houses, houses, bank loans, and new pages in our accounts payable and receivable books.

You see, it was like this, at least I think it was, though so much happened in those days some details now escape me. The big picture was my husband Hu wanting a ranch operation. I was ignorant of what this would entail but willing to support his wishes. Anyway, Hu could talk me into most anything. Oh, how I loved that enthusiastic aura of his. Everything seemed so reasonably do-able.

Though I have few regrets, I can't help thinking our lives would have been so different if we'd invested in an uncompli-cated lake cottage or even Canada Savings bonds instead of the ranches. No telling what trails Hu would have taken. But then I must remember that the need for land, cattle and horses was bred in his bones. What was in my bones? If I think hard, from my mother's family, an appreciation for beauty and civility, curly hair, and a distaste for confrontation. I don't think I got her strong will. From my father's side some quiet Irish humor, patience, small bones and curly hair. Only a few of these quali-ties helped me through the life of the Hidden Bar Ranch.

We called it the Hidden Bar Ranch, using Hu's Welsh vet-erinarian father's old cattle brand — HB (attached) with a bar underneath — a derivative of his name, Thomas Batin Harries. Tom Harries had a small holding out of Calgary where he kept his cattle. We were lucky to get his long unused brand in the family again, though we only used it on the commercial cattle and not on the purebred Black Aberdeen Angus. They were tat-tooed on their ears as is still the custom.

In the early years, every Saturday or Sunday we'd go from our own driveway in the city of Edmonton and head three-quarters of an hour east. The car would be cracker-crumbed and crowded. I'd have packed the usual picnic fare. As well, a box with a diaper bag, extra diapers, a dirty-diaper bag, wet washcloths, towels, rolls of toilet paper, extra training panties and overalls. Disposable diapers, like seatbelts and car-seats were still non-existent. I held the wiggling baby on my lap.

When we unloaded, the children raced or stumbled through the tall yard grass, then we all trailed after Hu. His face glowed. "That's where the new barn should go," he said, "and we can shore up the old one. And over there — a machine shed. We'll slash a lane through those woods to the meadow and have a small feed-lot behind the trees, so sorting pens can be here to the west. Great headquarters." His dreams and vision for Hidden Bar were visible only to him. I was as ignorant as the children.

Why can I envisage a ball-gown from looking at a bolt of fabric or a table setting when I pick flowers? I thought. My world was details. Not his, his was big picture. When I think about it, it wasn't as if he were a rich kid in a toy store, pointing and ordering whatever toy his little heart desired. But what do I know? After all, his family had had a farm and the first of his four univer-sity degrees was in Agriculture and we did have other income sources. Neither did I suspect then what the children and I would see and learn over the life of the Hidden Bar Ranch.

Hu could see exactly the future details of this property, while I somehow pictured something grander, more movie-like than what actually appeared.

It would take me many years to bask in the same quality of well-being that he must have immediately felt when he surveyed these acres of poplar scrubland. The land where small prairie sloughs and lakes were duck-splotched and beaver-damned. The land, many acres of it, was covered with poplar, spruce, chokecherry and wild rose, which was eventually cleared. It was bushwhacked and seeded yearly to make more pastureland for what became first a commercial herd of cattle then a herd of prize-winning purebred black Aberdeen Angus. We raised horses at different times — cutting horses, hunters and thoroughbreds. Thoroughbreds led us into the world of the racing back-stretch and involved us in a trucking business that hauled horses from the Atlantic to the Pacific, as well as a horse-van fabrication facility at the ranch.

There were so many purchases: fence posts, barbed wire coils, new wells, corrals, tractors, barns, houses. We were always one stage behind what we could reasonably afford while back in Edmonton, Hu was hustling in his economic consulting business and teaching extra classes at the University of Alberta. Our children, Bruce, Jody and Lori were growing out of their shoes, eating more and more. Jeffrey and Danny came along during more land purchases in the area. Our first son Tommy died when he was four, in 1953, the year of the big polio epidemic, the year before our first rural land purchase. Every September we worried there could be another polio plague.

Chapter 2

Harold was our first employee. We were lucky to have him help us start off in ranching since he'd lived in the area all his life. Not long after his arrival, his mother, Mrs. G. moved in with him. No one told us — certainly neither of them — but we guessed her husband was difficult and this was her escape route. At the time, I thought Harold's mother was old. She told me, "Eighteen years older than Harold," and I never knew his age, though I figured he was certainly older than Hu, who was nearly seven years older than me. So she seemed ancient. Today, I think she couldn't have been sixty.

Harold was a gentleman, handsome, lean and ever smiling. I think of him lifting our young children one by one onto old Penny's back and leading them, grinning, around the small corral in front of our first old barn. He would say, "Good for you — Penny likes you," when she would sneeze, jostling them into wide-eyed smiles. Harold's sisters were teachers who sometimes came for Sunday tea. Occasionally, I joined them while the men stood in the yard talking and the children played with kittens. I would caution Hu before I left, "Watch the kids don't fall in the horse trough,, though he did tend to be super safety-cautious.

We installed power, water and septic systems and a new electric stove and fridge in the small house the first year. "But of course we won't use the indoor bathroom in the summertime. We'll use the outhouse," said Mrs. G.

In those days, I was also answering nighttime calls from Edmonton constituents, since Hu had become a city alderman (councilor). In the city we needed plumbers and milkmen, babysitters and doctors, sand-piles and trikes and bikes and cough medicine and jeans. The ranch needed saddles and veterinarians and ranch hands and parts for tractors and oats and farmer's purple gas.

Harold suggested we hire Roy, an area farmer's son, since he was good with horses. Roy rode his horse — unless snowdrifts were too deep — back and forth from home to the Hidden Bar. His route was near where we cut our Christmas trees for home, school and kindergarten. It was where we had Hu's "arctic picnics." Parking the car on the highway's edge, Hu and eldest son Bruce broke trail and we'd slog through snow waist-high for the younger children. Then we'd gather firewood, pushing snow in a round high bank circling the large fire. One such picnic was always after Christmas when leftover turkey with *Lawry's Seasoned Salt* was warmed in an iron skillet and dropped into buns. I remember standing after I'd been sitting in the snow. My back was to the fire. I watched my little family, red-cheeked, gobbling the buns. Sparks from the fire rising and clicking in the early moonlit sky. That smell of cold, spruce bough fire and contentment will stay with me always.

Saturdays in the early days, when Hu wasn't traveling, he took Bruce, our eldest, with him to Hidden Bar. Bruce would be exhausted, too tired to eat, when they came home to town, always late for dinner. I would say, "Why must you stay so long?" And Hu would say, "We had things to do." Emergencies — broken water lines to the cattle waterer, a broken pump or they might have had to take a load of cattle to the stockyards. This would give Harold or Roy a weekend breather.

I teased Hu because he continued to buy adjoining land and other pieces. Finally we had three thousand acres. "It seems you always want the land next door. When are you going to stop?"

But with each purchase, everyday, freeze-framed details would etch in our memories. Scrubby poplars and willow inched next to the corrals at their east boundary. Gumbo in the corrals and the lane to the feedlot was lumpy with heavy hoof-prints. A tall manure pile in the center of the lot provided a vantage point where the animals would take their turns standing at crooked angles looking over the slat-boarded barn wood fence toward Antler Lake. The morning sun could seep through their tough hides and make them grunt, fart and moo with what could have passed for pleasure.

In summer, we found tiny strawberry plants in the old schoolyard. This grassy area was the field between the two-lane highway and our buildings. "Mummy, Daddy, here's s'more and here's s'more." They would be gorging, eating the tiny sweet berries, their faces, fingers and clothes stained red. I rarely had enough for full dessert bowls. While there was no sign of the old Uncas school, there was still the rusty school pump. Bruce and Jody were old enough to try taking turns pumping, but no water gushed forth.

I look at a drawing done by our six year old Lori. It shows Bobby, Roy's brother, who worked for us part-time, a red toque on his head making him look like a Santa's elf in profile. His arms are stretched forward holding the reins. He stands in the green wagon, the horses Mick and Flick, their manes shaggy, puffs of steam snorting from their nostrils in the cold fall air, their legs bending in peculiar ways. Lori draws the children hanging colorfully or peeking shyly from behind Bobby. Hay bales serve as seats and appear as squares of yellow, like blocks without alphabet letters. Each of the four children is smiling. (This picture was drawn before Danny was born.) A wobbling HB brand centers the wagon's side. Spruce and poplar trees fill the corners. The sun shines down. The sky is crayon-blue and cloudless. In a child's crooked printing is the misspelled "Hidden Bar Ratch by Lori Harries."

We had a weekend retreat at the edge of the woods next to the single men's bunkhouse — a faded red, second-hand trailer. It had only one bedroom for Hu and me. Jeff, the baby then, slept in a crib in the trailer. The other three children slept in the back of the station wagon.

Jimmy, a Calgary friend of Hu's, who had connections with some Stoney Indians, asked them to make us a tepee. The kids had great fun helping raise it each summer. Hu would yell, "Okay, up she goes," and Hu, Harold, Roy, his brother Bobby, and Bruce would heave on the long spruce poles slotted into the top flaps at the tent's smoke opening. Then he would say "Okay kids, let's see you paint some birds and buffaloes or whatever you want." And Bruce, Jody, Lori and little Jeff would push up their paint shirts' rolled arms, which were old made-to-measure shirts of Hu's. They had a size sixteen and a half neck, a forty-four chest and a thirty-six arm's length. The children used green and red barn paint to draw their own versions of native art on the outer walls of the teepee. There were camp beds with a fire pit in the middle. After hearing wails of distress some mornings, I would rush out flapping a tea towel at the magpies who strutted around the children's beds.

One awful day while Hu was away, Harold's sister Thelma phoned. "I'm at the University hospital. Harold lost his right hand in the grain auger."

It was terrible. He was with Roy, who applied a life-saving tourniquet. Each time we visited him he said, "I can't believe fingers that aren't here any more can hurt so much." Hu had insisted on a workman's compensation deduction from Harold's paycheque so he had a settlement that helped him buy his own place after he decided he could no longer work for us.

Chapter 3

I never did fit into that country scene. I didn't listen in on the party line, though my daughters did on occasion, so I didn't know which neighbors were ill or who had been in an accident. I didn't have a baby shower for a neighbor's pregnant daughter, didn't know whose daughters were pregnant, nor did I enter my wild blueberry pies or sprouted wheat bread in the local bake sale at the school. My cucumbers didn't end as crisp green fingers in jars with my own dill and garlic. I didn't know how to drive a tractor or operate the grain auger. Nor was I strong enough to throw a hay bale. I wasn't practiced in wielding a hoof-pick, a branding iron, a rasp, a welding torch or a post-pounder. What I did was help Hu and the girls do the scads of paperwork needed to apply for registrations for our purebred Aberdeen Angus cattle.

You see, I was a part-time rancher's wife, or rather, I was a full-time wife of a part-time rancher. We only lived at the Hidden Bar part of the summer: some weekends and occasionally during the week. Could I have become a citified interloper, carpet-bagging my way into a world of which I knew very little? I didn't know. In those days and later, I felt scattered enough as it was. Scattered as young mothers of five got in the '50's, '60's, '70's and '80's, with three ranches to visit, cook in and supply with, among other things, beds, bedding, tea towels, canned Danish bacon and mousetraps.

One of my extra-curricular activities during these times was to model in spring and fall fashion shows for stores in Edmonton. I would stride the ramps wearing the honest-to-God latest French, American and Italian creations, miles away from the Hidden Bar Ranch.

While the Hidden Bar increasingly played a larger role in our lives, what with the riding ring and the children's new-found competence handling cattle, horses, and farm equipment, I remained a novice. Mostly my place was in the kitchen. I was comfortable there and liked it, though sometimes I did feel left out. Of course there were those brief forays where I'd leave my post, trot to the pens, check off animals being weighed and loaded into large cattle liners. The snorting cattle would scramble up the ramp after being freed from a neck-squeeze apparatus. My fingers and toes would be numb while Hu and the children would be sweating — slogging through the corrals, waylaying and shoving the beasts into the desired locations.

So sometimes I was part of it. Part of the real activities of the ranch. But more often I readied meals, sat alone reading or took quiet walks into the garden, thinning the carrots, moving the hose, or gathering poppy pods.

Over time, the children and I developed a sense of place and affection for the Hidden Bar. In spite of the fact that I spent less time there than did Hu, I came to recognize its fine timothy horse hay, cattle feed and straw bales in the hay shed, its chicken coop with the pungent odor, the cattle and manure smell of the corrals and loading dock, the wonderful leather and horse feed perfume of the tack room, the heavy warm horse smell of the new box stall barn, the dusty air of the granary, the grease and welding smells of the machine shed. I also knew the direction the coldest wind would take. I knew the place on Antler Lake where ducks landed by the tall bulrushes and ruffed grouse ruffled their way across our paths; the place where my mother and I crawled on our knees on moss, picking the tiny blueberries of late summer which appeared in Sunday morning pancakes. I went to the Murray place with its sorting pens and sagging barn, where there were ink cap mushrooms that no one would eat but with which I made spore patterns on white sheets of paper.

We picnicked in crunching leaves next to a cattle trail, between one field and the next. In between were huge piles of poplars and spruce bulldozed and burned safely in the winter to create more pastureland.

There is a picture of us all, posed on bales in the hay barn. We used it for our Christmas card that year. It was Thanksgiving weekend. The sun is shining on our faces, warming the tough yellow-green strands of vitamins the horses and cattle would munch through the winter. Danny is the little one in the red shirt and black cowboy boots. He's three years old and watches his older brothers and sisters. Bruce and Jeff are wearing gum-boots. Hu may have had them tromping in the pens. I can't tell what Jody and Lori have on their feet. I wear a headscarf like the queen did when in the country, and sunglasses. Hu is smiling. Oh, he looks so young. He's probably thinking of how proud his parents would have been to see this sight. But also how worried they would be knowing the debt we'd tackled to have this place with all its cattle, horses and equipment.

It was young Harold B., a city friend of Bruce's, who took this picture. I can smell that hay shed. I can see the crows flocking. I can see through the leafless poplar woods into working chutes and beyond, the feedlot. Was it the day before Thanksgiving, when I would be thinking, what time will I need to put the turkey in the oven tomorrow? Remember to pick up whipping cream for the pumpkin pie on our way back into town.... what about those bank loans?"

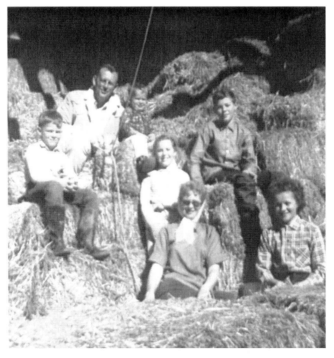

Thanksgiving — Hay barn — 1963

One summer in the ditch pond next to the home place gate where fireweed, Indian paintbrush and wild roses grew, we kept geese and ducks. Each night they were herded into a coyote-proof shelter in the barn. Budding engineers Jeff and friend Dougie built a wobbling dock into the pond. In the fall, the birds were shipped to a Kosher butcher who correctly slaughtered, plucked and delivered them frozen for our freezer, along with bags of their down feathers. I spent a day in my town kitchen dealing with this soft white blizzard. It still resides in cushions in my living room.

Chapter 4

Hu recognized hired hand Roy's quick brightness and encouraged him to go to university — the first in his family to do so. But before he went, inexperienced though he was, he began training cutting horses for us and had some small success. In those days there were not the half-million-dollar horses on the cutting horse circuit as there are today. Cutting is a sport begun by cowboys on ranches in Texas and Arizona which pits a specially bred horse named a quarter horse to cut an animal, a heifer or steer, from its herd — originally for shipping or maybe treating. The horses have strong hindquarters which enables them to stop and turn abruptly. In competition, the rider has two-and-a-half minutes to be judged on the success of the rider and the horse against the steer. So Roy left us to study Commerce at the University of Alberta where Hu was the Dean of the business faculty. While Roy was there they started a rodeo club for students and he married Greta, a secretary in Hu's economic consulting firm. During those years, a student told me, "I didn't think we'd live through it when the Dean quit smoking, his gas pipeline application was turned down, and his charcoal plant caught on fire." Those were just some of the ventures he tried in those very full days.

Bobby, who'd worked part-time for us through the years, replaced his older brother Roy. After he'd been with us a while, he married a local girl, Margaret. She was only about seventeen, I think. Never have I known anyone more shy than she. Like a fawn, she would lean into Bobby as though she could melt into him and become invisible. She would twine behind his slim blue-jeaned cowboy-shirted girth and Bobby would smile and say, "Margaret, what are you doing?" and she, eyes down at the grass, would say nothing. What did she think of us? Why was she frightened? When we invited them to a barbecue, after he'd gone to get their steaks, buns, salad and beer, she'd have him stand with her away from the noisy crowd. Then she'd hold her wobbling paper plate as though it might be sprinkled with strychnine. Bobby would smile all the while, adoring his tiny black-haired wife. I thought she looked like Walt Disney's Snow White. Maybe she'd start to smile and sing "Some Day My Prince Will Come." Although her prince had already arrived.

For two summers, Bobby and Margaret stayed in the red trailer and we had the little white house along with the new boys' cabin and girls' cabin for the older children and their visiting friends. These were roughly furnished with metal army bunk beds and nails in the walls for clothing.

We needed the larger kitchen since I became cook for three university students who worked for us putting up hay, fencing, feeding, and doing other chores. We had all our hearty meals on the newly constructed screened-in porch that hugged two sides of the little house. *Let's see, breakfast again today: dry cereal, orange juice, bacon, sausage, eggs, fried tomatoes, piles of toast, honey, crabapple jelly, coffee. What'll I pack for their lunches?* These young men lived in the single men's bunkhouse, which had electricity and a biffy in the bluebell and wild-rose wooded area behind. When we went away, Mrs. Sank, who had the general store on the way to North Cooking Lake, cooked for them.

Eventually Margaret became pregnant. When I asked when the baby was due she replied, "I'm not sure." I said, "Well what does the doctor say?" She floored me with, "I don't see him any more. I've kinda lost faith in him." Hmmf. I wondered what would happen. Nature took its course and they had a beautiful son. Two more children followed, all three strikingly beautiful. A few years later, Margaret began painting. Horses. Horses in profile standing on lawns with tiny flowers, and graceful trees drooping spring-green branches above their heads.

We always had our own dry-aged beef in the freezers. An appropriate animal was shipped to Mr. Gainer who custom-slaughtered and butchered the beast into too many roasts, steaks, stew and ground meat packages. We also began buying lamb from a friend in Lethbridge and Bruce and pals provided the odd small birds for our consumption.

One summer we had a field day for our friends. I had no idea what this would be like but, as usual, I was pulled along by Hu's enthusiasm. That dear man's yen for new projects couldn't be denied. And anyway, why would I want to? It was fun to go along.

Hu said, "You can't have a field day without a grandstand for the spectators," so he built bleachers on the west side of the riding ring. We invited friends with their children from town — about seventy-five as I recall. Roy and Bobby's uncle Albert brought some cowboy friends to do calf roping and cattle penning. For the kids there was calf riding and catching chickens in gunny-sacks, but only a few city kids wanted any part of these scary rural sports.

I provided the grub. I made many cartons of corn chowder which I took next door — very nervy of me, since I hardly knew Mrs. C. I'd only been in her home once before. However, in spite of many sponge cakes in her freezer, she let me wedge the chowder in for a few days.

After the excitement at the arena, the crowd had chowder, hot dogs, watermelon, ice cream, beer, pop and coffee. One of Hu's lovely traits was that he always told me how great the food was and what a success the party was, just as though I'd been in charge of the whole production.

During this period we had a shaggy-maned Welsh pony. Lori and her friend Wendy loved to decorate Miss Muffet with dandelion chains. Then they would take turns jouncing around the arena on her, laughing that she loved to wear flower necklaces.

One of those summers was when we had a pathetic orphaned calf, a Hereford whose expressive face was heart-rending. The poor thing was near death and seven-year-old Jody said, "Daddy, can I save her?"

Hu said, "I don't think so dear"

"But Daddy, can I try?"

"Okay dear, but I think she's too far-gone. You'll need to build her a pen, put bedding in it and then feed her with a bottle." So Jody gathered some scrap boards. One was an especially clean but heavy piece. She valiantly tried to hammer this across the corner of the nearest exercise corral in front of the new box-stall barn. The nails kept bending and it was hard for her to get it stabilized. Older, thinner boards were then applied. A final sign was nailed on: "Fawn." She brought straw and hay to her nursing station and called, "Daddy, I'm ready — can you bring me the calf and the bottle?" The patient and its nourishment arrived and Jody spent much of the afternoon coaxing the calf to drink while her subdued brothers and sisters watched. It was too little, too late and the calf died. There were many tears that night.

Andy, a son of friends from Toronto, came for a visit. He and Bruce became good pals, and Hu was attempting to get them all organized to saddle up for a ride to check fence lines. The boys were fooling around, as young boys do. Hu, the ever-cautious cowboy, shouted, "Andy, watch it — you don't know one end of a horse from the other." So ever after when Bruce and Andy set out on Squirrel and Rusty, Andy would grasp Squirrel's tail and say, "Want some oats?"

Chapter 5

We offered Hidden Bar for a three-day Pony Club rally in August, and prayed the weather would be as nice as it had been earlier, hot and with enough showers at night to cool things off and keep the grass growing. A rally is a huge undertaking. There would be up to one hundred people — parents and kids sixteen years and under with their horses and ponies from Alberta and Saskatchewan.

The world-wide Pony Club organization was formed by the British Horse Society to train young riders in all the correct methods of horsemanship.

Bobby and Margaret had left the ranch and Jim and Betty Lynn came to the little white house. Handsome Jim looked more like a high jumper than a cowboy. His legs were so long he looked like he could walk onto a pony from its tail-end. Betty Lynn was a glamorous Arabian horse breeder as well as a fine seamstress.

Hu and Jim spent many weekends before the Pony Club event with three knowledgeable couples, a number who were riding instructors and whose kids were active in the movement. These other couples all knew far more about the English riding scene than we did. Our children didn't yet have the horseflesh or knowledge to compete. Although they were thirteen, twelve, nine, eight and four, only daughters Jody and Lori poured over the red, blue and black Pony Club textbooks filled with instructions, data and lore about horses and horsemanship and dreamed of the day when they too could take part in a rally.

The two girls and their three brothers eventually did compete in horse shows, using the Pony Club books as backup.

I thought, *these people all know so much about horses. They talk more about horses and ponies than about their children.* Two of the women became district leaders in the movement and another developed a distinguished career as a jump course designer, traveling the world and hobnobbing with royalty at horse shows.

At first, Hu, Jim and these Pony Club experts hiked through our fields, took down fences, moved rocks, fallen trees and old rusted equipment and began building safe but challenging trails and jumps. One of the more exciting jumps was called "the piano jump." It began at the top of an outcropping, and came down, one "key" at a time— a challenge for the young competitors. Our cattle and horses were driven to the farthest corners of the sections. This was in order to build an interesting cross-country course. The rally was to be a three-day event, like at the summer Olympic games. Friday through Sunday events included cross-country, stadium jumping, and dressage classes.

Jim tilled the muddy arena next to the old schoolyard with sand and wood shavings to make the footing stable for the stadium jumping and dressage classes. We converted barns for visiting ponies including the old cow barn we used as a veterinary hospital in winter. It was cleaned out, its manure hauled to distant fields.

That barn had once housed the three-nostrilled calf that Lori and Jeff were going to take to a circus to make their fortune, although it died before they could put their plan into action. The kids did their bit too. They helped clean the tie-stall barn, and readied the new box-stall barn with straw and water buckets. The girls housecleaned the tack room and converted the machine shed into a stable with straw and buckets.

Hu outfitted his personal crew (Bruce, Jody, Lori, Jeff, four year old Danny and me), with big paintbrushes, red barn paint and assigned us to the new unpainted bleachers. I remember him calling out, "Come on gang, I've got an important job for all of you." Fortunately, we more or less completed that project before the teeming rains hit.

Under threatening skies and then pouring rain, borrowed Imperial Oil bunkhouses, arranged for by one of the Pony Club dads, were set up. Porta-Potties were put in place, a chow-wagon and dining tent with tables and chairs were set on the grassy area by the red trailer, next to the single men's bunkhouse.

The first of the three days began and I remember seeing a line of yellow slickered silhouettes snaking through newly flattened grasses on their way to the turquoise biffys. I crossed my fingers that the sun would come out again. We didn't need this.

Finally we began. The P.A. system called out the classes before the events. Parents' hearty good humor attempted to help their velvet-helmeted young riders keep their concentration for the trials ahead. Thank goodness the dressage competition, somewhat like ballet on horseback, and the stadium jumping could go ahead safely because of the good footing in the arena. There was some worry about the slick sloppiness of some of the trails and areas on the cross-country course, but the intrepid young riders came through safely. I have no recollection of any extra accident insurance or parental forms absolving any of us in the case of disaster.

When the whole weekend came to its soggy end the cheers suggested it was a success. It took a few days to return our horses, cattle and equipment to their former spots after the bunkhouses, chow-wagon, tent and biffys disappeared, and ranch life returned to normal.

Some time after the rally, Hu started riding a cutting horse, Birdwell's Tex (Tex), while Bruce rode Toby for a couple of seasons. Hu really enjoyed the new sport and we had commercial steers available so had many competitions at the ranch.

Most of the times Hu went to contests in Calgary, Vancouver and small towns across the province, I went with him. What was really fun was at the Douglas Lake ranch near Kamloops, B.C.

Because he was away so often, or busy at the University or consulting office, he didn't have the time to devote to the sport as did a number of the other amateurs, many of whom were retired men.

As for me, I recall one year I was unable to stop reading Nancy Mitford books, while Hu warmed up his horse in-between events. I thought of my life and how different it was from that of the crazy Brits in those old orange and black Penguin books, "The Pursuit of Love" and "Love in a Cold Climate."

Chapter 6

Before long, the children needed ponies and horses and velvet riding hats and britches and tweed jackets and boots and saddles and cowboy boots and spurs and more Pony Club books and boxes of elastics for braiding horses' manes and tails and snaffle bits and halters and bridles and saddle soap.

And Hu produced three rodeos in Toronto at the Maple Leaf Gardens and ballpark. The first was a financial disaster because customers were hunkered down at their televisions watching the Kennedy assassination clips. The other two were better, though they were also financial drains.

At the house in town, I kept two sets of seven pairs of jeans washed and wrestled onto metal frames to dry. Denim in those days was not stonewashed and soft. By the time the jeans were comfortable, they were on my mile-high mending pile next to my sewing machine, which I left open on a counter in our bedroom. I constantly broke needles going over the GWG, Lee Rider or Levi heavy seams.

Then we bought the Stampede Cattle Station — fourteen-thousand acres of southern Alberta prairie grass with five farm-steads, many employees and purebred Aberdeen Angus cattle.

After doing a successful economic study for a German Steel company, Hu was asked to be the chairman of its Canadian board and we went to Dusseldorf for meetings.

Before we knew it, the kids needed hair dryers and lipstick and nail polish and Beatles records and ballet, riding, guitar and piano lessons. We worried about drugs, motorcycles and dirt bikes, while our horse trailer-trucks and the hitch of eight heavy show horses gobbled money faster than the bucking barrel in the main ranch yard regularly tossed riders into the sawdust.

When Jeff was fourteen we sent him to Calgary to take a course enabling him to do artificial insemination on our black purebred cows. By this time, we'd bred a very high-class bull, Byergoes Black Revolution, and along with expensive vials from other bulls, his semen was regularly used. Jody and Lori spent summers at Stampede Cattle Station riding the many miles, detecting and penning cows for this procedure.

In 1968 at the Hidden Bar Ranch we built a four-bedroom log house complete with dishwasher, swimming pool and boys' and girls' cabins. It was in this house where we had our Saturday and Sunday brunch parties, offering omelets cooked to order. One year I made raised pork pies which I vowed I'd never do again. It was too nerve-wracking. Crazy. In those days, we nearly all smoked and at these parties drank Harvey Wallbangers, which were vodka and orange juice with a float of Galliano. It was always bright and sunny, though cold. Our guests crunched crookedly down the driveway for home as the sky turned pink in the west and the sun lowered.

In early summer, our kids always had their high school grad breakfasts here. Parents chaperoned and cooked bacon, sausage and pancakes on the outdoor grills. Of course, everyone fell or was tossed into the pool before changing into bathing suits, and the dryer whirled.

This was also when Hu began commuting to Ottawa for the four years (1968-1972) he was a member of parliament under Pierre Elliot Trudeau. We bought the Paradise Ranch on the shores of Lake Okanagan in British Columbia where we ran a unit of purebred cattle and then turned some of its silted cliffs and orchards into vineyards. I worried about Hu. How he could keep up the pace. We were, of course, ever more heavily "into the banks."

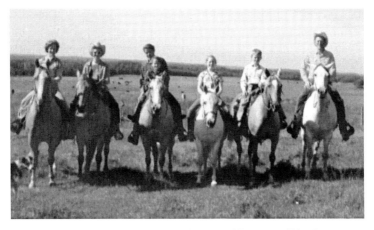

Jody on Flora, Joyce on Mocha, Bruce and Danny on Toby, Lori on Snow Goose, Jeff on Sundown, and Hu on Birdwell's Tex

*   *   *   *   *

When Jim and Betty Lynn moved on, we built a yellow bungalow next to the foundation of the original settler's cabin and Albert and Gail came to stay. Two sons were born to them at Hidden Bar and they brought some of their relatives, Ronnie, Frankie,

Jim and Gary to work through the years for us at Hidden Bar and the Stampede Cattle Station.

Hu was traveling abroad for the World Bank and we bought the large church place (formerly owned by the Mormon Church) at Hastings Lake with its half-section hay meadow dammed yearly by beavers. Roy became an expert at dynamiting these dams. He'd worked for us years before and had left to study Commerce at the University of Alberta while Hu was the Dean of that faculty. In the winter, Albert used heavy horses and a sleigh to feed the cattle, which was a more reliable method of feeding than a tractor-pulled breakfast.

Twice, we went to Aberdeen Angus World Forums. First, in Aviemor, Scotland and next, to Christchurch, New Zealand where Hu gave a paper on I-can't-remember exactly-what, but I recall that it was well received. Great trips, purebred cattle, and fine people.

Eventually, most of our wells at Hidden Bar produced hard water, which magically turned scotch a gray-purple color when Hu poured drinks into large glasses for visiting cattle buyers. I knew there would be suppressed grimaces after they saw the expensive brown bottle tilt, and what happened after, when Hu poured a small amount of water into the scotch.

This was all at the log house — from 1968, until 1981 — the end. I call those years the biggest, the busiest, the best and the worst years of Hidden Bar Ranch.

Chapter 7

I know I was a necessary part of the team. In the kitchen of the big house, I prepared soup, not salads, roasts, not pizzas, stew, not stir-fries. In the long spring days, when Saskatoon blossoms frothed next to pale green leaves, and frost had almost melted under three feet of manure in the pens by the loading dock, I set meals on hold and walked down to the action station where Hu's voice rose above the mooing grunting of the animals and his shouts, "Get over to the side Bruce...Jody, not that way, towards the fence...Lori, Jeff, Danny...look sharp."

Only occasionally would I have a task at the pens. Perhaps recording weights as an animal stood on the jiggling platform of the weigh-scale, or counting the critters as they were admonished physically and vocally to clamber up a ramp to a cattle liner, their snorting, farting protests unheeded. When I think of it now — the sounds, clear as rolling drums and the smell of heat steaming from winter-coated bodies and manure plopping on newly thawed gumbo. I'd watch a driver leaning against a front fender of his well-kept truck, cupping an ungloved hand around a sputtering match as he lit a cigarette. Our burly veterinarians, either Dr. McLean or Dr. Klavano, cheerfully stating, "Well gang, that's it for today," and I'd trot back to my kitchen.

One winter morning when we came from town to the ranch we drove through the main yard and saw the heavy horses leaning as they often did, against the metal pipe corrals. Vapor from their nostrils and steam from the water trough clouded the area next to the red pump house. Its motor labored on this minus-twenty day. Hu said we had to ship two loads of purebreds to Virginia and the vets had to clear them.

At the main house I turned up thermostats for the two gas furnaces, which were kept on low setting while we were away from the unlocked ranch house. Everyone except me climbed into grubby snowmobile suits, Sorel boots, woolen toques and down mitts. Hu said, "Come down after a while and see how we're doing." I thought, *he really wants a coffee/hot chocolate delivery.*

I recall looking out the large kitchen window at the woods. Trees and bushes surrounding much of the backside of the log house were poplar, pine, high bush cranberry, chokecherry,

Saskatoon and wild rose. That weekend, they'd all been touched with a double-sifting of snow. It wasn't a damp heavy snow like in the spring, but rather more like icing sugar wafted from a sieve on a fancy dessert. I wondered what the Inuit name for this kind of snow would be.

Later, in two trips, I took lemonade thermoses, now filled with hot cocoa, two other giant thermoses of coffee, mugs, a sealer of milk and jar of sugar along the cleared road to the corrals. My boots made scrunching sounds and bits of snow dislodged from branches as the occasional sparrow went for vitamins stored in the few remaining frozen berries.

I saw the bawling cattle, shaggy and unkempt looking and thought, *poor things, they're sad.* No longer were they the shiny oiled specimens I'd admired a few months earlier at the Toronto Royal Winter Fair. I knew the heifer, winner of Best in Show, was no longer here. Nor did they look as they used to when they munched grass in their summer pastures here and at the Stampede Cattle Station. Cows were often trucked to Stampede to calve out in the dryer, earlier spring.

I hung around while Hu, the kids, Albert and the vets sorted, tested, then pushed the snorting animals up a slippery chute into the liners. It took time.

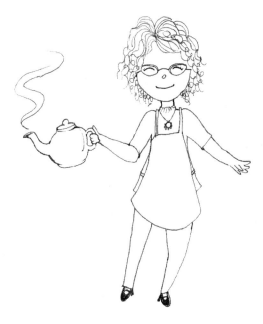

Before they finished, I hurried back to my kitchen where I turned up the heat under the soup pot, took the plastic wrap from the platter of cold cuts and cheddar cheese, plunked the jar of dill pickles on the checked tablecloth, made a big Brown Betty pot of black tea, glugged milk into the dark green plastic pitcher, and set out the plates, cutlery and mugs. Lastly, I buttered the buns, putting them in brown paper bags to warm in a very low oven.

I could hear them approaching the back porch, which we'd cleverly made from used though smelly creosoted railway ties. The mudroom door burst open. Cold air blew into the kitchen. Thunks and clunks. They took off their boots. The toilet flushed again and again. Taps turned on again and again. And they trooped in, laughing as usual, and squished in around the table. I stood in the working area, making more and more tea.

This had been my role, and I was not discontented. When I look back, nearly forty years later, I thought then those were only snippets of solitude. I now recognize that snippets of solitude were and are, gifts.

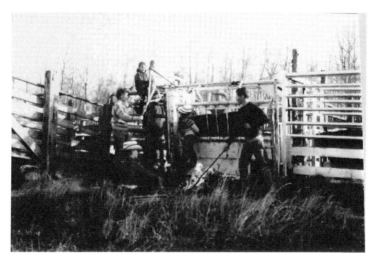

Branding day at the squeeze with the whole family — 1964

Chapter 8

Some weekends when we moved cattle to the northeast corner of the Hidden Bar, I'd take the yellow truck to the Bennett corner to meet the cattle and riders who'd maneuvered south to the tricky turn into the Murray place. I'd seen what could happen if a few bouncing black cows took it into their heads to keep going south instead of going through the small opening to the lush northwest front field of this property, which was separated from our home place. Those maddening critters would jounce along like an ink blob. They'd stay on the road or ooze along fireweed-filled ditches, tails swinging, running like crazy, as though they had one internal compass among them. One animal would do something foolish, perhaps end at a small holding with a barking guard dog, and suddenly they'd turn tail, troubled and wheezing, doubling back on themselves. I'd stand in the middle of the road, arms and legs spread, yelling "yo…yo…yo," thinking, *this sure beats peeling potatoes for stew.*

I'd watch as our mounted company — cowboy-hatted, leather-chapped and loud voiced — whistled and put the spurs to their horses. They'd round up the errant beast and push it back through the correct gate to the herd. Then they'd move up the lane into the mustering pens by the old Murray barn. I'd drive the truck through the fence opening, wrestle with the gate, almost in tears, thinking, *fee-ble, fee-ble. Pull harder.* My boots sliding as I leaned back, hands holding the loop of heavy wire to slide over the post-top. Finally, the gate of wobbling saplings wrapped with barbed wire went from limp to stiff in the closed position. With a satisfied grin, I'd jump back into the truck thinking of the lunch jouncing in the back of the pick-up. If I was a proper rancher's wife, we'd have homemade buns and apple pies.

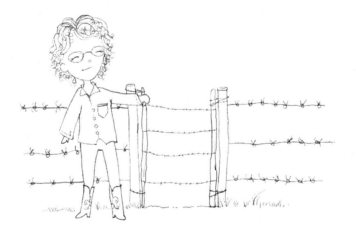

One year, late fall, when it was too cold, we had a purebred Angus sale at the ranch. For publicity, we offered proceeds of one calf's sale to the Edmonton symphony. That attracted the Edmonton Journal who sent a photographer and writer. Hu installed large portable space heaters in front of the sales area by the big hay barn.

An idea of mine to warm up the buyers and put them in a better bidding mood was to provide hot stew with buns and hot mulled wine. These were to be sold. Coffee was free. The idea was that Jody, Lori and I would make kettles of this stuff. From the profit the girls would reap enough money to put towards a ski trip. The boys helped in the pens, which at least kept them hopping and warmer than the shivering buyers who stood with hands in their pockets. My plan ran fine, except it was difficult toting the stew down to the pens and I hadn't allowed for a heat source there. The cattlemen didn't like our sweet lukewarm wine, preferring to pour their shots of liquor into the free hot coffee (which we had made in rented coffee percolators). Our catering profits were zilch. But the cattle sold. We didn't repeat the effort the next year and went for private sales only, as well as continuing our yearly sales at the Stampede Cattle Station during Calgary Stampede week.

Then, on the way to Banff, where Hu was to attend directors meetings for the Banff School of Advanced Management, I remember him saying, "I know, why don't we put a small subdivision on the ranch? Leave the home place with houses and everything. We'll put a new road in from the main north-south road." As usual, he had the whole plan in his mind.

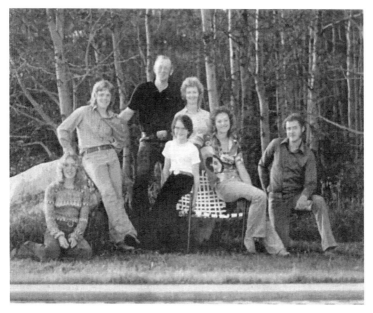

At Hidden Bar Ranch: Lori, Jeff, Hu, Danny, Joyce, Jody, and Bruce — 1971

Chapter 9

After two years negotiating with the local planning board we finally got permission to develop a subdivision called Farrell Properties. It was named after my dad. I chose and ordered six pre-fabricated houses and sited them. I was adamant that kitchens face east to get the morning sun (on acreages you can do this). Bruce and his friends Brian and George, who could operate a backhoe, set the foundations. Bruce hired the carpenters. I contracted for the floor coverings, appliances and hired the painters.

Oh, the problems I had with Pat the Irish painter who too often didn't complete a job when he said he would. I'd heard that many painters become alcoholics and I wondered about Pat, but had no reason to think this was why he didn't show up when he said he would. I furnished one show home without spending a cent. I used an office desk covered with floor-length cloths for the dining room table, borrowed beds, pictures, a chesterfield and chairs and put many dried flower and grasses in corners–the style in those days. When one show home sold, I moved the furnishings to another.

Many years later, when I was a florist for the designer of show homes, I found myself thinking, *no wonder only buyers with special vision purchased our spartan acreage properties.* At first, most weekend open houses were under my command, but we finally turned this job over to real salesmen. Our goal was to sell these six acreages with houses so the remaining properties would be more saleable. And, over time, they did sell. I thought that was the end of that.

Well, it was, until we decided to develop another piece of the land. This site bordered the west side of Antler Lake, its southern boundary running partly along the main line of the C.N. Railway. To counter objections from the Planning Board that houses might be too close to the tracks, I visited eight households whose homes were located even closer to the trains than the ones we had planned. Those householders told me they, "Just love the sound of the train's whistle at the Uncas crossing. It's a comfort!" When I asked if their dishes fell out of the cupboards when trains rumble past, they laughed and told me, "No." They heard the trains as we did–a song familiar as geese honking overhead in the fall, coyotes yipping throughout the year, and frogs croaking in springtime.

I remember the final hearing that granted us permission to tackle this project. Hu sat between me and Kim, who was the town planner we'd hired to design the Antler Lake Meadows. When a witness spoke of the possible inconvenience of the railway tracks being too close to some of our acreages, Hu disagreed so heartily, Kim and I each put a hand on his knee, pressing hard, to keep him from jumping up and objecting. In the end we got approval.

Fortunately, we built the roads and sold the whole project just before a drop in the real estate market. It helped with the banks, but we were still overextended by their twenty-plus percent interest rates.

Then Albert and Gail left to start their own ranch and we knew they'd succeed. It was because of Albert's quiet competence and Gail's red-headed energy. Succeed they did. Many years later, Jeff's eldest son, Hu, spent part of two summers at their ranch, learning about a place so different from his family's vineyard home in the Okanagan.

That spring we also celebrated a family wedding in Edmonton when our daughter Jody married Jan. The beautiful bride wore my wedding gown remodeled for her more curvaceous figure. Her glowing sister and three grinning brothers were all in the wedding party. No blue jeans.

Chapter 10

We had a series of incompetent employees after Albert left. One was a thief who stole Hu's best trophy saddle and also Jody's Steuben English saddle. Neither of them was ever recovered. Then Koski came to us from Japan with his wife Myumi and little boy, Kazu. They stayed until the end of the Hidden Bar Ranch.

One day, the machine shed caught fire with both Koski and Hu in it. Hu said he saw the blue flame snaking along the ground to a tractor, and yelled, "Koski, get out of here *now!*" They ran out separate doors just before the building blew up and threw them into the air. One leg of Koski's jeans was alight so he rolled in the grass. Then he ran to the corrals. Hu ran to our house shouting, "Get Billy up from his nap. The place is on fire."Fifteen minutes later the county volunteer fire department arrived. By this time flames had destroyed the garage and shed containing Hu's valued restored '28 Chevy and '49 Mercury trucks plus two snowmobiles, tractor tires, grain auger and oat storage, and I-don't-know-what-all-else. Flames leaped not only across the road to the large metal building where we fabricated horse vans but also to the metal corrals behind. They didn't reach barns or the hay shed. Koski and Hu drove the cattle and horses to safety.

I had grabbed our dozy little grandson, whose Mummy was in Ontario, put him in the truck's passenger seat and drove a short distance away from the log house. I can still see the outcome — the smoke haze and little Billy sitting on the fire engine drinking apple juice.

A neighbor took Koski to the hospital for treatment on his one leg. Thankfully, there were no other injuries to humans or animals. Before this I had been visiting my mother daily in hospital, and this was the only day I didn't visit her, six weeks before her death.

This was about the time that Lori caught the 'cutting horse bug' and often went with her dad to competitions whenever she could. Hu did well on Doc's Twister. Lori ended up as the Canadian novice rider champion on Mia Freckles.

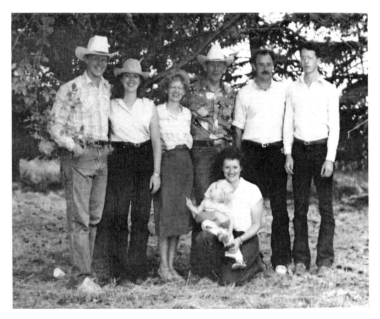

Family at Stampede Cattle Station on Sale day — 1978

Chapter 11

How did it end? It was spring, when poplars cast their char-treuse haze and ditches were full of spring run-off. Hu left the office early. We arrived at the log ranch house, and Gyp, the ranch dog, panted alongside the car from the barnyard and through the trail to the log house.

Through the car window, Hu called, "Glad to see you Gyp, you run pretty fast for an old fellow." I took the basket of dinner extras from the car while Gyp's feathery tail waved around me. Early evening sun shone through the wooded west edge of the clearing at the back porch. Hu said he was going to check with Koski and would be back in a while.

So quiet. I knew Hu had been thinking how different it was now that it was just the two of us. I didn't mind, but he must have seen the writing on the wall.

I lit the barbecue and basked in the early evening glow. Crows were cawing and gophers were popping in and out of their holes. Horses stood at the fence-line in the front pasture wondering why I was just standing there, doing nothing. But I was thinking. Thinking of this place. Thinking of how much longer we could hang onto it. The place where we'd started the whole ranch scene for our family. I felt it couldn't be much longer. The children were rarely here. We'd sold the Stampede Cattle Station in the south, and we'd cut back on the numbers of purebreds. Though, as Hu patiently tried to explain, you need volume. Now we could concentrate on the vineyards in B.C.

I made a salad, cooked a sirloin steak, tented it with foil, and, before dinner, Hu poured us each a scotch. We sat staring at the tall fieldstone fireplace. I smiled, "You were so glad when you finished building it."

He frowned, then smiled. "Wish I'd had time to help with the stonework. Nice to think, isn't it, that the stones are all from our own fields?"

No TV or radio. We talked about the children, the future of the Paradise vineyards, what the future held for us, and what was right and wrong with the world.

We sat at the old mahogany dining room table, sun striping across its dusty surface. I'd run a tea towel across it but the results were not perfect. I'd put a few short branches with bursting leaf buds in the speckled pottery vase. I felt a tear. If the children were little, this would be filled with dandelions.

Hu leaned back in his chair. "We have to, you know. Sell. What do you think?"

"I know. It's time. We still won't be free of the banks, will we?"

"No." He reached over and took my hand. "We'll be over the worst dear."

We would sell Hidden Bar. Have an auction. A land auction, the first of its kind in the area.

And so, Hidden Bar was sold. June, 1981. I stayed for most of the day in the house. I could bring myself to watch cattle going under the hammer. But this? Our home-away-from-home? Where our children had come every summer and many weekends. Where ranch-hands, truckers, veterinarians, Mounties, politicians, foreign students and dignitaries, local university students and professors, scientists, cutting horse contestants, cowboys, European board members, Hu's economic consulting staff, relatives, friends and neighbors, high school grad party groups, all had sat at our tables, drank tea, coffee, beer, scotch, wine, cokes and hot chocolate. They had eaten rare and over-cooked steaks, beans, corn chowder, hot dogs, hamburgers, wild blueberry pancakes, made-to-measure omelets and my one-time pork pies. This ranch was where our children had learned to ride horses and drive cars. Where they'd shot skeet with their friends. Where all the kids put ponies over jumps, learned the odd ways of horses, cattle and chickens, and the ways of people from various walks of life.

I listened to the faint sound of the auctioneer's loudspeaker, background to my thoughts: *Hu must never think this has all been a big mistake. After all, many of his dreams became our dreams. It's been quite the education for me and the children. And I love him for it.*

People who work sitting down get paid more than people who work standing up.
— Ogden Nash (1902-1971)

*The above story can also be found in Athabasca University's Alberta Women's Memory Project, under "memoir collection."

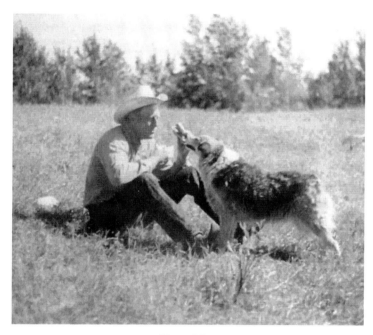

Hu and Gyp

The Almost-Original, Three-Onion, Three-Cheese Casserole

Does this ever happen to you? You get a deal on onions (or some other basic item). Two bags for the price of one. The other day I bought two and got two free. Quite a few onions for one single woman. But never fear. *I can do this*, I thought.

I Quisinart-ed them with a slicer blade, without too many tears, then caramelized some of them. Of these caramelized ones, I used a few spoonfuls on a leftover beef patty for lunch. Next, I divided some of the slithery onion mass into freezer bags. The rest were for the required onion portion of a casserole — to be cooked in my white oblong enameled iron pan.

The recipe called for three kinds of onions: yellow, red, and leeks, three kinds of cheese: Havarti, cheddar and Boursin. I made double the recipe to take to the Royal Tomato Society weigh-in. I knew my tomato was big, but was unlikely to take the prize for the heaviest, but I did have a medium sized specimen that was so grotesque, it was bound to win the most ugly category. For the dinner, I had to take a deliciously different vegetable dish. It didn't have to contain tomatoes.

On the same shopping trip, I bought bags of peppers to start making my sweet and sour pepper jelly. Every fall, without fail, I can't stop myself — I make this jelly. I'm down to eight decorated jars from last year's efforts. I use these for hostess gifts as well as on my own table. Corn was twelve ears for four dollars and I bought six. I slightly tweaked the casserole recipe by adding chopped red and green peppers, cornrows cut from the cobs and lemon thyme. This last item was from my autumn garden. I'd already harvested most of it, which was drying in a brown paper bag hanging from a hook over my kitchen table. Even with a doubled recipe, I only needed one cup of white wine, and since it seemed silly to open a bottle for just one cup, I sipped a glass while I put the dish all together. I planned to have a friend over the next day to finish it off. The recipe said to cook for one hour, which was not quite long enough, since you want the onions soft, not only limp. I still had some yellow cooking onions left, but they're good keepers. I'd bought too much Havarti cheese but that'll get used and I couldn't bring myself to use two packages of Boursin because of the price. So I substituted cream cheese light for the second Boursin package, and added fresh parsley and dried tarragon to it. I found that it worked to halve the amount of melted butter and spray the casserole with a light Pam instead.

The Almost-Original, Three-Onion, Three-Cheese, Casserole (changes as above)

6 portions
- 3 tbsp. unsalted butter
- 2 large yellow onions, thinly sliced
- 2 large red onions, thinly sliced
- 2 medium-sized leeks, (instead of sweet onions). Well-rinsed, dried and thinly sliced
- Salt and freshly ground black pepper to taste
- 1 ½ c. grated Havarti
- 2 5oz. package Boursin cheese with herbs, crumbled
- 1 ½ c. grated Gruyere cheese
- ½ c. dry white wine
Preheat oven to 350 degrees.

Butter an 8-cup baking dish with 1 tbsp. of the butter.

Make a layer in the baking dish, using a third each of the yellow onions, red onions, and leeks.

Sprinkle the layer lightly with salt and pepper. Top with the Havarti and make one more layer of the onions and leeks, seasoning each with salt and pepper. Top this layer with the Boursin. Layer the remaining onions and leeks and top with the Gruyere. Dot the top with remaining 2 tbsp. of butter. Pour the wine over all.

Bake for 1 hour. Cover top with aluminum foil if it gets too brown. Serve immediately.

> **There is no love sincerer than the love of food.**
> — George Bernard Shaw, 1856-1950

Handbags — Then and Now

I was fifteen in 1943 and sometimes saved a partially smoked cigarette. I butted it when it seemed expedient, and shoved it, warm and unsafe in my bag, to be extracted and re-lit when the coast was clear. My pint-sized black patent leather bag also held a brown cloth change purse with a two-knob metal closure. It contained green street car tickets, a paper shin plaster worth twenty-five cents, a brown two-dollar bill, two humbugs in wax paper twists, a greasy Tangee lipstick (orange in the tube and pink on the lips) and a Tampax tampon (new on the market). The bag also held two ironed hankies, one with the initial 'J' and the other with 'Monday' embroidered in blue pink and yellow, although it wasn't Monday.

This purse contained a half-used turquoise-and-white package of Kool cigarettes and matchbooks. These were small free packages of matches advertising places such as the Silk Hat Restaurant on Jasper Avenue. The Silk Hat served mostly French fries, grilled cheese sandwiches and raisin pie a la mode. Tea-leaves were read there by a succession of angular women, their long earrings swinging in the smoke-filled air.

A round, lace, zippered evening bag matched my first formal dress, both made by my mother. The dress's skirt was white-dotted net, its bodice navy blue crepe with a white lace ruffled sweetheart neckline. Years later, the white net skirted our first baby's bassinet.

Another evening bag made by my mother had circles of yellow eyelet dyed to match a yellow pique summer evening dress.

Evening bags were, and still are, intended to hold a minimum of gear: lipstick, comb, perhaps a pressed powder compact with mirror, tampon and hankie. Money, called 'mad money,' was a requirement.

When I was much older, I needed a larger purse. It was loaded with Dinky toys, arrowroot biscuit crumbs, records of immunizations shots, a card reminding me of the date of my next obstetrician appointment. I'd transfer this appointment onto the white and blue I.O.D.E calendar hanging crookedly by a string on the wall next to the telephone on the kitchen counter above the toy shelf. This bag held a fountain pen needing an ink refill, a pencil needing sharpening and one black glove; the other one was who-knows-where. There were no rubber soothers in my bag, as they were frowned-upon in those days for being unsanitary. A partial package of Player's cigarettes was lodged with a silver, initialed lighter in the purse's depths.

Later, my purse kept boarding pass stubs. No cigarettes. Lists like, "pick up Hu's suit, get skates sharpened, guitar strings," or, "elastic for ballet slippers, birthday gift, Tues., Mary, Jody, shoulder pads to dressmaker," or, " deposit cheque, Montreal," (A cheque from one bank to be deposited to cover an overdraft in another bank in those heady days before instant communications). As well, in those days, there were evening bags, one made to match the black velvet gown I loved.

Now my purse is always a shoulder bag. In its deep, dark bottom, at least five round, white-and-black, medium tip, easy-to-hold, BIC pens without their caps, only two of which are loose in the purse bottom, along with a small ring-binder for notes and thoughts to myself. In a side pocket, a half-used package of Halls honey cough-candies, a small package of Tums, a small pocket-calculator, a business card holder, a lipstick in a holder with a mirror, extra house, garage and car keys. My wallet is loaded with more sales-slips than cash, coupons for Air Mile points, and special offers. My purse also holds sunglasses, glasses-case, two red leather gloves, one rumpled worn-thin lace-edged hankie of my mother's with a slight tear in its center, a folded hard copy of an aging joke about a woman reading in her husband's fishing boat and my eight-by-five inch diary book, which helps me keep track of my appointments, messages, phone and other important numbers.

Now I change between winter purses and summer purses. I have evening bags some thirty years old, one I needle-worked to go with a taupe, cream and metallic gold sweater I bought in Toronto when we were 'flush.'

"Not my purse…the only way I know I exist is if I have my stuff with me," I overheard an attractive woman at the next table say. The man she was with had asked her, "What can you do without?" I doubt it was the answer he was looking for.

Today, bags are sought-after as style statements. Buying bags has become a fixation for flocks of females, taking over from the shoe craze. My lunch companions want knock-offs of the latest 'It' bags — anything Chanel, many-pocketed Marc Jacobs, Prada, Kate Spade, Hermes, Birkin or a Fendi Spy. Stylish types look for bags that don't show phony or real logos, thinking they will be judged trend-followers. Instead, they look for that supreme specimen that could go with almost everything they own; just as a man wants shoes that will do the same. The bag must be supple, and sturdy enough to hold much of their lives. It should look French, Italian, nonchalant, and whimsical all at the same time. In short, an impossible purchase. So, she finds the nearest thing to perfect and continues hunting for 'The One.' Bags pile upon bags on her shelves.

There are handbags, evening bags, shoulder bags, disco bags, clutch purses and pocketbooks. Many evening bags are based on designs from a more opulent era. They can be soft or hard-sided with only enough room to hold a lipstick, hankie, credit card and cash. Many evening bags are art pieces costing far too much for the usefulness they provide. They contribute to a long list of items modern women crave, but can't have.

> *Remember that the most beautiful things in the world*
> *are the most useless: peacocks and lilies for instance.*
> —John Ruskin, *The Stones of Venice,* 1851

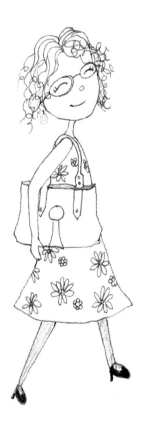

Surprises of Widowhood

While the ambulance siren wailed, we wove madly between construction barriers on a main highway. The red-faced, sweating medic, whose eyes met mine then slid away, told me without words that his efforts to revive Hu were going to be impossible.

There were no widow warnings for me before, or on that day; August twenty-six, 1986, two weeks after my fifty-eighth birthday. I've since pondered which is worse: to have a beloved die with no warning before one's eyes, or to have him linger in pain or befuddlement, you soothing as best you can, agonizing over the inevitable.

The past often loses its chronology. Time jerks backward and forward. My memory stops like a clock run down to the day he died in front of me in a strange town, while riding his horse, Doc's Twister, in a competition. That day, Hu got his wish to die with his boots on.

I'm surprised each time there is a flashback, prompted by some convoluted connection. It might be prompted by hearing Aretha Franklin or K.D. Lang, or by reading a newspaper headline, 'Are Politicians to be Trusted?' I might think of it when a daughter phones, a horse whinnies, a son phones, or a grandchild rings the doorbell. I think of him when I see a headline, 'Gas Pipeline from Alaska,' hear a radio report on more scholarships for first year university students, catch a re-run of *Fawlty Towers*. When I hold a new grandchild, or an older grandchild drives me to the airport, when it's apple pie season, or a bulldozer pushes a pile of trees, I think of him. A headline,

'Was Shakespeare the World's Best Writer?' a large white bath towel, Joy perfume, at least a dozen red roses in a vase, Wales, all of these remind me of Hu. Maybe the scenes associated with these prompts are not real because Hu isn't here to confirm the accuracy of my memories. I think, *if only he could see or hear or taste or smell this.*

I was grateful, and not surprised, when, following Hu's death, my friends brought food and their concern for our children and me. When one is a widower, what's known as "the casserole brigade" of lonely women continues to minister their good cooking upon the grieving single male for many months following his wife's death. This was not necessary for me.

I was surprised when a group of about a dozen anonymous women friends gifted me with an all-arranged surprise holiday in Arizona. I traveled with a friend from another city, who'd been one of my bridesmaids, to visit another friend in Arizona. We'd been her bridesmaids. Then I was sent to visit old friends who'd been my neighbors for thirty-eight years. After that, I visited another friend whom I'd known since I was thirteen years old. This was some time after Hu died; after Lori was diagnosed with M.S. After I'd been selling my products at farmer's markets and craft shows. Before I ran artists and writers retreats in the Okanagan and before I started writing.

I didn't grieve for Hu in a publicly dramatic way. It isn't in my nature. I didn't go through the great anger stage, which is supposed to hit all grieving widows. Finally, I realized I could smile instead of cry when I thought about Hu. I loved him for the way he treated me. He was a romantic. Was never mean. He called me *Little One*. I loved his amalgam of sentimental, tough, smart, sensitive, inquisitive, enthusiastic traits. I've been watching my adult children, looking for the same traits in them and in their offspring. Although I'm sure I would have done this even if their father/grandfather hadn't died.

A woman I didn't know well asked, "Have you recovered yet from your husband's death?" She said it with a concerned look and tone of voice and I'm sure she meant well. I said, "I'm not sure, I think so."' She said, "It must be easier if you had a good marriage than a bad one."

I mumbled, "Yes, thanks." I've thought of this often. I think she was very perceptive and I wondered what her life was like.

It isn't surprising, now that I am getting older and more reflective, that I think about the difference between grieving for our young child, my parents, or my husband. There is a difference. At least there is for me. Sometimes it's the same, only different. It took me a long time to recognize the cruelty of having to say goodbye to our little boy in 1953 when he was taken from the ambulance to polio quarantine and surgery and six hours later our doctor appeared at the door with, "We lost him." We only had four and a half years to get to know our first son. I grieved more for what we were yet to experience with him than what we knew at the time, although this observation could very well be incorrect hindsight. As for my parents, both gentle presences in my life, I was relatively young. I was forty-two when Dad died, and fifty-three when Mother died. Each of them gravely ill in hospital, one with a severe stroke, the other a brain tumor, their deaths were releases. I was left parentless with no siblings, feeling the weight of being at the "top of my family." I am now older than either of them were when they died.

I've rarely spoken to other women, an increasing number of whom have joined the widows' club, about some of my whirling thoughts on the topic of widowhood. Oh, once in a while something comes up that's appropriate, but much of what I think about is particular to me and Hu.

I keep coming back to the fact that Hu is now twenty years younger than I am. When he was alive, he was the "older man," wiser and nearly seven years older than me. It's confusing. Not only am I now older than my husband, but also, on some days, my children attempt to trade places with me, making me the child and they the parent.

A few years after her dad died, daughter Lori, on hearing I'd accepted a dinner date from a man I'd met in a Tai Chi class, said, "Do you know who *he* knows? Be sure you leave a phone number where you can be reached. Don't drink too much wine and be sure to not stay out late." Really. She needn't have worried, and might have known, no one could take her dad's place.

Then when I told son Bruce I'd talked during a play's intermission to a man sitting next to me, who'd invited me to a lecture on diamond mining in the north, my son said, "Don't go Mom. He probably thinks you're a wealthy widow." Which I'm not. "But if you do go, don't sign up for any diamond mine shares." In the fullness of time, this man's company was competing for diamond pipes with DeBeers of South Africa, and its shares zoomed.

After I'd moved to a new house, I couldn't imagine Hu living in it. It's too small. He'd be okay sitting in the kitchen at the east end of the table, on the L-shaped banquet, holding a phone to his ear and laughing, but what about the university student who stays with me and keeps me company at breakfast every day? I'd be making breakfast for two men. The upstairs bathroom shower and our bedroom would be far too small. Hu's Italian silk bathrobe hangs on a hook on the back of the bedroom door next to my bathrobe, which he has never seen. Once, when son Jeff visited, he wore his Dad's robe, startling me, his long leg-bones and his feet so like his father's. Hu would hate the computer desk and all the papers and files and the lights on the fax, which glow green at night across from our bed. Our bed; the same double-extra-long where we planned and conceived four of our six children. The winter quilt is different, as is the summer bedspread. The pillows have been re-downed and a new thin foamy sits on the quilted, sagging blue mattress. Pictures of our children as babies and young-sters line one wall. Above the closets filled with my ancient and newer clothes hang university graduation pictures of our five children, seventies and eighties hairlines on the boys and still an innocence in the girls' smiling eyes. Where would Hu's shirts, suits, ties and blue tracksuits fit?

I was used to Hu's absences. When he was away in our earlier married years, we wrote and latterly, unless he was abroad, phoned at least once a day, so I heard his voice. He always asked to talk to the children. After he died, when the phone rang at night, I'd reach for it, and think, *it's him.* I'd feel his presence, but before I'd touched the receiver, he was gone. Somehow, he was absent and present at the same time for that instant.

A man I didn't know well said, "You are now the matriarch," and a picture came into my head of a smart woman in black telling her adult children and grandchildren how they must conduct their lives. I would think, *What a fraud I am. I can't do this. This family needs a patriarch. Hu would have been so good at it.* I still think this, though of course his role wouldn't be that of the suave manipulator of my momentary dream.

*   *   *

I didn't know their names. He shuffled and she took short steps. His neck needed a trim, and the seat of her slacks was droopy. The sidewalk was too crowded to pass, so I walked behind them impatiently, but noticed their hands were clasped. And I thought of Hu, my long-gone man, holding my hand when we first blind-dated to a movie at the Capital theatre.

When we walked the hospital corridor to the viewing window of the maternity nursery, we held hands while gazing at our first child, and our second and third and fourth and fifth and sixth. Then later, when we walked to the rink to see our children skate, the back lane icy, he held my hand. He held my hand when we followed our eldest son's coffin, November sky gray and low.

And when we walked that last hill together, Okanagan silt puffed 'round our feet, we swung clasped hands, looked at the mountains, heat-hazed and hot. His hand large though fingers talented enough to fix watches or write speeches and essays.

I wonder, if he were still alive, would we two be holding hands, shuffling and short-stepping down the avenue, an impatient widow on our heels?

*   *   *

August. The month of warm days and cool nights. My mother used to say, "There's something in the air. Yesterday the air changed. We're going into fall."

Hu would say, "Ethel, every August you say that and it shortens summer."

But she was right. I felt it when I opened the stair-landing window on my way to bed. It's my birthday the day after tomorrow and three days after our sixty-fourth wedding anniversary. Four family birthdays this month and in a little more than two weeks, the anniversary of Hu's death. You'd think, twenty-six years later, I wouldn't still feel a physical yearning as though even one touch of him could make this disappear.

I'm surprised when a friend tells me I was very brave after Hu's death. I wasn't. There was no choice.

Now I know I've moved on. I have friends who didn't know Hu and I participate in activities he never would have dreamed I would.

I was surprised the other day, in the middle of a street, when the new pedestrian lights tick-tocked the seconds I had left to cross. I raised a bare arm to keep my straw hat from flying off, glanced at the inside of my lower arm and couldn't believe it was mine. Fine wrinkles like a plum left too-long in the fruit bowl, had appeared. Surely this condition had struck me overnight. What would Hu say?

Today I sat on my east patio with my legs in the sun. I was reading and drinking ice water and I thought all of a sudden, *life is good. Remember this day. When winter comes, remember how you feel — somehow eager — though for what I don't know.* Perhaps just eager for more life. I'm not too hot. The tomato plant behind me is doing its best to enlarge the fruit before season's end. I crush tiny leaves in the V of some of its branches and the fragrance remains on my fingers, perhaps transferring to pages in my book. The sky is clear blue. This morning I had a good interview about my book for a university catalogue and a phone call out of the blue from a man who'd read my books and said I was brave to write them. He told me he had appeared often in court with Hu and admired him.

I'm not surprised that while I look at the past with mostly a smile, remembering, and remembering, I can also look ahead. More great-grandchildren, family and friends' companionship, family weddings, travel, books, and more writing.

I've come to a point where I can ponder the sweep of my life so far. But I can't help thinking, *not yet, but oh, I hope I die like Hu did while doing something I love.*

> **There is absolutely no substitute for a genuine lack of preparation.** — Anonymous

Good humour is one of the best articles of dress one can wear in society. —William Makepiece Thackeray

On reading a report that the smell of lemons evokes feelings of generosity and perhaps significantly reduces crime rates:

The Smell of Lemons

should a lone woman
out walking late at night
carry a cut lemon
in her bag
the better to
improve moral behavior
in case a predator
pervert
latch his beady eyes
on her
she will sense his stare
finger her lemons
not to squirt as he pounces
but to wave the cut fruit
in front of his nose
the purity of its perfume
will stop him
morality swirls
he changes his tune
smiles
good evening
nice night

Ice Wine Grape Harvest at Paradise Ranch (No Wonder Ice Wine is So Expensive)

Come with me to four nights in mid-December in the year 2000, to the Paradise Ranch near Penticton, British Columbia in Western Canada, at the north end of its most southerly vineyard, the Koosi Creek.

I'm wearing borrowed felt-lined boots, a down jacket, ski pants and silk underwear, warm gloves, a wool toque and scarf. In spite of this, I shiver and stomp my feet. I need to get to work — then I'll warm up. I'm amongst 100 other warmly-clad people waiting for 20 acres of grapes to feel the effect of a dip in temperature (minus-8 to minus-10 degrees Celsius). These special grapes weren't picked during the fall harvest, and have managed to remain out of the clutches of deer, elk, bear and birds. They hang in leafless splendor until they freeze, concentrating their sugars. We won't begin picking until the grapes have reached a tested hard texture. Then they'll be pressed into concentrated juice, which gets turned into the ambrosial nectar called Ice Wine.

Searchlights are on hoisted on trucks — theatrical lighting for us since we're important members in the large cast who produce Ice Wine. Lights, forklifts, trucks of big and small bins are positioned at one end of these Riesling grape rows. We fan on either side of the trellised rows, our small bins on the frozen ground under the lowest wire. I taste the green-brown grapes, which become sweet sherbet on my teeth and tongue. We squeeze our sharp clippers, dislodging the marble bunches hanging prolifically from their vines, and they fall into these bins. A skiff of snow has polished the slopes to slippery slides. When our bins are full, we pull them down the slopes and dump them into larger bins. Forklifts load and unload these 800-pound bins into the huge press, which extracts the precious juice from the grapes. This juice is then siphoned into large stainless steel vats for fermentation and further alchemy at the winery. A full moon above Campbell Mountain shines bright white. The drivers of both forklifts and trucks go faster, slithering on the icy trails. One almost goes over a cliff. The temperature is now minus-12 degrees Celsius.

Many of the pickers are from the East Indian community around Penticton, their heads and mouths swirled in colorful cloths. One of them, temporarily across from me (we work either side of the trellised vines) asks, "Where are you from?"

"Edmonton."

"Why are you here?"

"I'm Jeff's Mom." "How old are you?"

"Seventy-two." And he turns to the muffled figure next to him and speaks in a language I can't understand, although I hear the name *Jeff* and see the message relayed down the row as far as I can see. I wonder if by the time it reaches row's-end, I am a miraculous 102.

At midnight I go down the hill to bed. I dream of grapes with wings, flying to the loading dock where they magically roll themselves into the press. In the morning, I'm told the temperature dropped to minus-14 degrees Celsius. I hear the bad news that at about 3:00 a.m. one of the press' functions ceased. The other pickers, who had by this time completed the harvest on the lower plateau of Riesling, were now well into the heavy crop of Chardonnay. They are told to go home. This harvest night they will not see that magical coming of dawn, when the pale cerise light creeps from behind the Douglas fir-covered mountain spilling its warmth down the slopes, perhaps halting the harvest. I am told the press can be fixed. Now if only the weather will co-operate and stay at least a frigid minus-8 to minus-10 degrees Celsius. Already I understand why there are only 350 Ice Wine producers in the whole world.

The next night, we're at the Salish Trail vineyard, in the Merlot grapes. These grapes are a dusky-red lipstick color and have a grapier taste than did the Riesling. This vineyard is on the northern end of the Paradise Ranch, in a high half-bowl facing south. Searchlights beam toward it like a rock concert at Hollywood Bowl. Eighty-five of us pick until 4:30 a.m. when we move back to Koosi Creek to the Chardonnay. These grapes are pale chartreuse. It's hard to separate their bitter seeds, and I eat a few, whole.

In November 2000, the Paradise Ranch 1998 Chardonnay Ice Wine won a double gold medal at the 2000 American Wine Society's Competitions (this means all judges placed it first) and its '99 and '97 Chardonnay Ice Wines won gold. In February 2001 their 1998 Chardonnay Ice Wine won a bronze medal in France at the Chardonnay du Monde and in April 2001, it won the Gold Medal at the VinItaly International competition in Verona, Italy. It's well known in the wine industry that Canada is the world's largest producer of Ice Wine.

The next night, 'though below zero-degrees Celsius, the temperature doesn't reach minus-8 degrees Celsius, so we can't pick. So I go up the hill and watch the grape-pressing process. It's been going on around the clock, as it will for seven days after final harvesting. Men have flung bright orange thermal blankets on waiting bins to keep the cold in. I watch these men and marvel at the effort and stress that's involved. After all, Ice Wine, just like good perfume, is a very special concentrate. Neither is exactly a staple of life, nor are they inexpensive, but oh, they both titillate the senses more subtly than any other substances I can think of.

It's now the last night of the Ice Wine harvest and at 7:00 we're back at the upper Paradise vineyard in a block of Riesling. The first two rows show heavy bear damage. There, the poor bunches have only a few withered raisin-like nobs on their twisted stems. A picker next to me says, "I was told that last year a herd of fifty elk ate 10 tonnes of grapes just before harvest." I wonder what the bear tonnage losses are. We move on, clipping and dumping, clipping and dumping. I unwind my scarf and take off my toque; I must be moving faster tonight, I'm not the least bit cold. Overall at harvest's end, 135 tonnes of grapes are put through the press.As I pick, I think about the lucky people who will someday gratefully sip Ice Wine made from these grapes. Will they pair the small glasses of precious fluid with a pâté and a side of apricot chutney? Or perhaps they will try it with a creamy blue cheese and a sliced ripe pear? Will they roll their eyes, smile and say, "We must do this more often?"

Over a bottle of wine, many a friend is found. — Yiddish proverb

Resting with a View

I walk through the back door of the ancient flat-roofed house, past gnarled old apricot trees, then the garden. The corn is only a bit higher than my waist. Next, I walk through the old horse barn inhaling its smell of manure and saddles, then through the chicken pen, past clucking bronze and white hens and one manly rooster. I skirt the base of 'the pyramid,' a hill without tombs, but dotted with wavering old cattle trails, pale mauve field-orchids, sage, and the echo of grandchildren's piping voices.

Then I stride through the horse pasture, where two ponies raise their heads from the lush grass, swish their tails, then return to their grazing. An alert coyote stands on an overhanging bank, his ears cocked, tail stiff, creeping Oregon grape at his feet. I wrestle a wire gate open, go through, close it and go across the old hay meadow to a clump of wild plum trees. Browned fruit on the ground is mushed into tall pink-and-white sweet-smelling clover, timothy, and purple vetch. Fresh bear scat tells me who has been here for a feed.

I puff past the hay barn, now sheltering lengths of old irrigation pipes, snakes, and mice. Elderberries, green though tinged with purple, lean against the barn. My knees are beginning to hurt, but I go up the rutted, dusty road past rows of Riesling and Sevel Villard grapes, around the bend where Lombardy poplars we planted twenty years ago stubbornly hold the edge of a gully from sliding into the bay. Then I hook around to the left, past the first of the thorny blackberry bushes dusted with tractor-generated Okanagan silt, and go uphill through the rows of Vidal grapes to a bench area. Pioneers planted plums here, and perhaps their seeds were carried downhill to the meadow sixty years ago. Now, short rows of Riesling grapes guard the rock-ledge trail to Merlot grapes, large ponderosa pines and a private graveyard (not ours). The graves are marked only with stones. Occasionally, a bright orange tiger lily pokes between the pine cones and needles blanketing the ground.

A breeze lofts from the lake below, ruffling the edge of my straw hat. I walk around the stone markers, thinking about those who are sleeping forever on this high promontory. I look up at the cloudless sky and across the lake to heat-hazed mountains where ashes scattered to the Okanagan winds will alight one day. And I think of others, in other graveyards–somehow, some way, their spirits whirl around me. I am dizzy with my thoughts.

There is more to life than increasing its speed.
— Mahatma Gandhi (1869-1948)

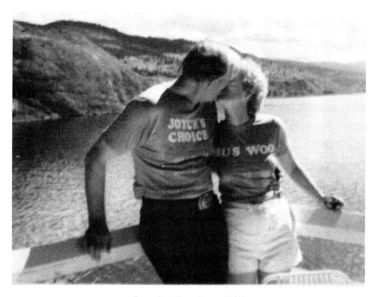

Paradise Ranch — 1975

— *117* —

I'm Going to Paradise

when lightening strikes
and sends me back
I'm going to Paradise
in an orange dune buggy
Okanagan winds toss clouds of silk
I'm going to Paradise
on one side
cliffs of butterscotch fudge
the other
ponderosa cones rattle
I'm going to Paradise
cherry trees with sparrows
wasps in apricots
geese honk on shore
minnows dart
milkweed pods rattle
I'm going to Paradise
swallows in machine shed
spot white on tractor hood
vines push grapes to bunches
a horse whinnies sage brush
powders under sun's scorch
I'm going to Paradise
but where are the people
they are there
barely there

I can see each one
hear them laugh
they look at me
through me
oh where am I
where is Paradise

Poetry is when an emotion has found its thought and
the thought has found words. —Robert Frost

Who Knew What

Certificates from both the London Cordon Bleu Cooking School and the British Horse Society and Pony Club set Bridget apart from the other two au-pair applicants I interviewed in London. Besides, her attractive English accent reminded me of a younger Greer Garson in *Mrs. Miniver* and I thought her calmness could bring sense to our obstreperous daughters. Like Beth did in *Little Women* or like Olivia de Haviland, playing Melli, did in *Gone With the Wind*. They might stop using slang. I may have been carried away, but this time in London at the Savoy Hotel with Al, without children, had mellowed me to the point of fantasizing. She'd be a sensible older sister to our girls.

What had struck me about Bridget was the openness of this barely five-foot tall twenty-year old was her firm handshake, and most of all, her background and obvious willingness to move to Canada. "I'm sure you'll fit right into our family, Bridget."

She arrived at our ranch on a hot July day in the mid-sixties and early the next morning, she appeared in white shirt, beige britches and high black boots. We were off to a horse show in a small town where we asked her to keep an eye on our youngest child, four-year-old Jackie, who wasn't riding in any classes. The other five ranged from seven to fifteen, and needed both my husband and me to help them prepare for English and Western classes. Each time I glimpsed Bridget she was grooming a horse or playing with kittens in the barn or talking to fifteen-year-old

John, as he towered handsomely above her on Sundowner. She didn't appear to be actively babysitting Jackie. He played nearby, sweeping, and running his tiny trucks through wood chips spread in the alley in front of the stalls. At four, he was accustomed to avoiding much of the manure. A hot sun intensified the overall odors Bridget was used to at her mother's farm in Kent. I'd read somewhere that upper-class English females were more interested in animals and men than they were in children. I hadn't thought of this when I was interviewing her.

Bridget became my competent extra pair of hands and when we had a dinner party, she was our built-in caterer. When I traveled with my husband, she cooked, shopped, drove the kids, and followed my long lists attached to our kitchen calendar.

Our two eldest, John and Ann, quite liked Bridget. Often, when Al and I came in before midnight on school nights, we'd find the three of them giggling and drinking cocoa in the den. When Al asked, "What's so funny?" the answer was always, "Oh nothing Dad."

Since our new resident didn't have a social life with people her own age, I suggested to the eldest son of neighbors that he take her to a movie. He passed the honor to a friend who owed him a favor. The next time I saw Don, I asked him if his friend didn't like Bridget since he hadn't asked her out again. Don grinned, and said, "I'll tell you about it some day." I looked at him quizzically, but left it at that.

When I asked, the morning after the big date, Bridget said, "He's a nice boy." I didn't give up on my efforts to socialize our little Brit. Before Christmas, the family had a meeting and decided we'd give her a ski-week at Sunshine Village in the Canadian Rocky Mountains. She deserved this treat. So, bundled and starry-eyed, away went our English rose on the Greyhound bus for what we hoped would be a blissful time away. She returned wind-burned and smiling but rather subdued. I put this down to exhaustion and carried on with my own whirling life: helping my husband with our travel agency business, running two houses, loving and overseeing six children.

Two months later, over our usual late afternoon cup of tea, Bridget confided in me that she was pregnant. I felt sick.

"I drank too much hot mulled-wine after a big day on the slopes — met a couple of American students. There was a roaring fire. I didn't feel well, and then it was morning."

What to do? She said she wanted an abortion. *Whew.* Remember, this was mid-sixties. I couldn't imagine aborting any of ours. I'd thought, *how awful,* but I didn't know her family situation at home. Should we bring her through a pregnancy and encourage her to place it up for adoption? I sent her to my obstetrician but she would have nothing to do with an abortion, as I knew she wouldn't.

*   *   *

That night, when Al was almost asleep, I whispered, "It's all my fault." "Mmm...yes dear."

"So naïve — damn hormones — but if we'd never sent her there, if she'd stayed home with the family, she'd have been safe."

Bridget phoned her mother in England to see if she could arrange an abortion in Sweden. We didn't tell the kids why, but the next week she left, with the whole family long-faced and me in tears.

What would I do some day, if Ann, Margaret or Nancy came to us with this story? When I didn't hear from her, I phoned her mother. She told me that Bridget had aborted the baby the day after she arrived in England. Her manner was aloof. She said that for the last few years Bridget had been a bit of a problem and she'd hoped the girl would cool down living in a completely new setting such as ours. She thanked me and said

Bridget spoke of us with great affection. I wondered what this cooling problem of Bridget's could have been. She seemed healthy: good hair and skin, good physical condition. She never had a cold. I had no problems with her temperament, nor had I noticed an over-abundance of energy.

*   *   *

Forty years later, I am a grandmother many times over and my children are raising teenagers of their own. We gathered as usual after Christmas dinner in our long living room. We always show old fashioned black-and-white home movies. Reels and reels of them. There are always pictures of the first day of school, riding two-wheelers for the first time and many reels of horse shows. Our eldest son, John, runs the projector backwards sometimes as he has done since he was seven-years-old. He has children walking backwards up stairs, bicycles pointing frontwards though traveling back, and numerous ponies jumping nimbly, though backwards, all this for grandchildren's hilarity. A frame appears with Bridget leading Margaret's white pony, Ghost, and I said, "Poor Bridget, we've lost track. Wonder what's become of her…that pregnancy…good she lost it."

My adult children gasped, "Mo-om…she what?"

"Well, I know we didn't tell you then, but didn't *one* of us mention it — in forty years?"

They rolled their eyes, said, "No-oo", and Ann said "Mom, we used to spy on her. We walked the top of the fence next to the hired men's cabin at the ranch and looked in. She came on awful strong." And then the clincher: "And Mom dear," her voice became gentle, more incredulous, "When you were away, she was always after John."

I looked over to where John manned the ancient movie projector. The film usually landed at some point in a slithery heap on the carpet. Not this year. Tick, tick, tick, tick, tick, tick. The film gave a final flicker and his hand turned the off knob.

'Tis not every question that deserves an answer.
— Thomas Fuller, *Gnomologia,* 1732.

The Tidier Years

It's not like when my family was young.

I think of our back hall — winter in the early sixties. The window above a counter splayed with schoolbooks is iced in a swooping line along its lower edge. Outside, the snow falls, feather-like. Pillows of it empty all over the land.

Hand-knit mittens are clothes-pinned to hangers on hooks to dry. Their wet wool fragrance is a winter smell as definite as the baking potatoes and meat loaf in the oven. Every light in the old house is blazing. Streetlights are on and the children have tumbled in for dinner from their after-school tobogganing and skating. They all talk — shout — at once. Their voices mix with the smell of cold. (I believe there is such a thing.)

The older two, Bruce and Jody, noses running, moan, "We're starving."

Lori crosses her legs, wails, "I have to go to the bathroom,"Jeff announces, "I can skate backwards!" Little Danny lies on the floor whimpering, "Mummy — help — snowsuit — off."

It had been peaceful for almost two hours. The porch door is wedged half-open as snow has clogged along its hinge-side and cold seeps through the milk delivery door. Puddles of melted snow from moccasins and over-boots shine on the dark green linoleum. Two hooked mats are askew and skates and jackets are not quite hung.

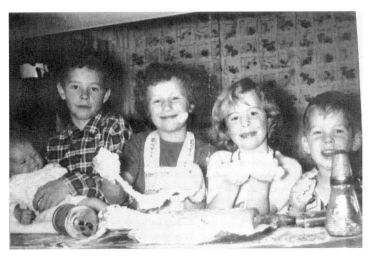

Baby Danny, Bruce, Jody, Lori, and Jeff making Christmas cookies — 1960

Today, in my sedate, but not senile years — the tidier years — I look at my small front hall. My jackets and coats from all seasons fit on one pole. The shelf above holds book bags and winter and summer hats, including that sweat-stained cowboy hat worn by Hu when he died in 1986. And next to it, the funky tweed hat he wore that day we were in Wales when he posed for my camera in front of Llwyn-y-Groes. This was the deserted stone farmhouse his father left before World War One. He'd come to Canada as a fifteen-year-old to seek his fortune in Canada. I remember how Hu grinned at me, and how pleased I was that the hat didn't shade his face for the picture. Somehow, that roll of film didn't turn out, so it's now a mind's-eye memory each time I fling a scarf or bag high onto the shelf.

A broom and a shovel lean into the jackets. Next to them, my safely — treaded, zippered boots are placed side-by-side. Wet spots on the mat under them show I've been out recently. The small porch, steps and sidewalk to the road are clear. I'll let someone else do the main shoveling job. Snow fell in the night and a marshmallow glob of it sits on my round patio table.

Son Danny's coming for dinner. It *can* be baked potatoes and meatloaf, though, more likely it will be stir-fried chicken or micro-waved fish with lemon, both with rice. Funny. My tidier years have brought changes in my kitchen and in my menus. My bread now comes, fragrant and crusty, though from a bread machine. Teflon coats my meat-loaf pan and pepper is in a grinder. A red wok receives fresh ginger and garlic before cornstarch-coated chicken and vegetable shards. A radio and CD player are on the counter, and my tiny kitchen's floor is covered in blue-and-white speckles.

Now I can sit and read if I want or watch TV while dinner cooks. Not like the years when I was sometimes so frazzled by five o'clock that I'd have the older children watch the younger ones while I escaped to a bubble bath in our long green bathtub. I would read a *Good Housekeeping* magazine and try to ignore sad pleas from a little one leaning on the locked bathroom door, " Mummy — Mummy — Mummy."

It is quiet. No need for a bubble bath now. I hear only the purr and click of the furnace through the vent under the sink and the hum of the fridge motor, its small freezer crammed with leftovers made into dinners-for-one.

A version of Ann Lander's Meatloaf

Serves 6

- 2 lb (1 kg) lean ground beef
- 2 beaten eggs
- 1 ½ c. (375 ml) breadcrumbs
- ¾ c. (175 ml) ketchup
- ½ c. (125 ml) warm water
- 1 ½ gram pkg. (45 g) dry onion soup mix

- 1 tsp salt (5 ml)
- ½ tsp (2 ml) pepper
- 2 bacon strips
- 1c. tomato sauce
1. Preheat oven to 350 degrees.
2. Mix everything together except bacon and sauce.
3. Pat into 9x5 oiled loaf pan.
4. Lay bacon the length of loaf and pour sauce over it.
5. Bake one hour.
6. Rest ten minutes before slicing.

Microwaved Fish

Serves 2
- 2 mostly-frozen fillets of fish — same thickness.
- 1 lemon or lime (for juice and rind).
- Knob of fresh ginger, peeled and finely grated.
- Oil spray
1. Spray glass pie pan
2. Place fish in pan.
3. Pour juice over it, then sprinkle rind and ginger over all.
4. Cover with bowl or paper towel.
Cook for 4-6 minutes, full power.
5. Remove from oven, check for doneness. If necessary, cook longer.

Chicken Stir-Fry

See p. 143, 144, "A Woman Who Cooks, Eats and Talk About It"

> *There is no such thing as a little garlic. Good to eat and*
> *wholesome to digest, as a worm to a toad, a toad to a snake,*
> *a snake to a pig, a pig to a man, and a man to a worm.*
> — Ambrose Bierce (1906 The Devil's Dictionary)

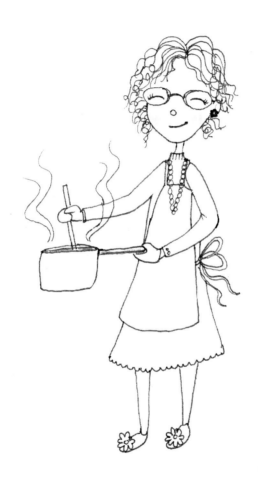

Melting Time

There must be *something* in it. I just heard it again today. This time from a woman I've known for five years in a writing class. I've always loved her stories. She's eighty-three and claims, "I can take pasta, rice or pizza a few times a month, but I need my meat, potatoes and vegetables."

My cousin tells me her mother, my aunt Marjorie, whose one-hundredth birthday we celebrated three summers ago in Victoria, was only content with a meat and potato dinner. My Aunt Floss on the other side of my family lived to ninety-five eating meat and potatoes with butter (no margarine) and was still making Christmas cakes a year before she died.

My friend Mary, the one who prompted these thoughts, had just given me a generous slice of her fruitcake kept moist with a piece of sheeting soaked in brandy and apricot liqueur. A month-and-a-half ago she had made twenty-two pounds of this luscious dark fruitcake, divided into four cakes. My sample was from the fourth. The other three cakes were to be decorated by a caterer and tiered for her wedding— her first — to a man she had known and loved fifty-three years ago, though hadn't heard from in thirty-five years.

This past spring the man, Doug, happened to talk to Mary's sister-in-law and found out what his long lost girlfriend's life had been about. He remembered how they had met after the war. He'd been discharged from the RCAF, was at university taking agriculture while she was in education specializing in English. They'd hit it off and eventually had an "understanding."

Then they had a fight that escalated into one of those situations where neither could back down. They parted and went their separate ways; he to farm, and she to leave the small one-roomed country schools she'd formerly taught in to take her place at a large composite high school in Edmonton.

When she moved to the city, she encouraged her many nieces, nephews, grand-nieces and grand-nephews to live with her while they went to university. Sometimes these sibling offspring numbered one, though more often, there were multiples of up to five in her home. At the moment, one niece and her three children and one nephew are with her. She tells me she's counted all these young people, their spouses and offspring and the grand total is seventy-four. She says these young people have been wonderful to her through the years. I'd say they were a lucky lot to live with their Aunt Mary.

Doug, her long-lost boyfriend, wrote to Mary suggesting they might reconcile. She was stunned at the suggestion, still holding to the idea she never wanted to see him again. (Of course I was discreet enough not to ask what their fight had been about.) She threw his letter in a drawer where it languished for six weeks. She thought, *This is not being very Christian. I should at least be decent enough to answer.* So she sent him a cool note in return, he phoned suggesting they meet for coffee. They met, after which she invited him home for lunch. They spent the remainder of that day talking and fifty-three years melted like butter in a fruitcake.

When I said, "Mary, I hope he's a nice man," she replied, "He's perfect."

She has asked me to do the flowers for their wedding. She says Doug likes roses, so I've ordered two kinds of white and a pale peach. On Sunday I will go to my floral wholesaler to order the remainder, to be picked up Thursday morning. She showed me the bridesmaid and matron-of-honor dresses in lavender and blue and said, "Of course, I'm wearing white."

Quarrels in France strengthen a love affair, in America they end it. — Ned Rorem, *The Paris Diary of Ned Rorem* 1966

The Late Queen Mother and Me

When I'm one hundred years old, will I wave genteelly from a balcony to cheering crowds? Or will my children and grand-children gather for the biggest birthday party of their lives? When I'm one hundred, will I have a daily gin and Dubonnet, as the Queen Mum is said to have downed for the last we-don't-know-how-many-years? And will I be comfortable wearing Cuban-heel shoes made to match my outfits? Will I wear hats with flowers or feathers whenever I'm out in public? Will I have badly tea-stained teeth? Will I walk upright, except for canes I must lean on, due to recent hip surgery? The Queen's good bone density is probably due to all the milk she's consumed in her daily Scotch porridge and in her tea. Oh-oh, I rarely eat porridge and I drink my tea clear.

Will I be thinking when my one hundredth comes, *Why am I still here, when so many young have died?* Or will I be thinking that straight at one-hundred-years of age? Will I play the races? I know I'll no longer be a thoroughbred owner–haven't been that for years and wasn't ever committed to it as the Queen and some others I know are. Never got past the "claimer" category and didn't study bloodlines and "form" as the Queen did. Nor did I place the same hours of attention to bloodlines and char-acteristics of Aberdeen Angus cattle, as she did. At the time we were in that scene, her ideas about the breed had become "old-fashioned," while we were on the cusp of a flourishing Angus specialty world.

I was never an angler as she was, wearing hip waders and standing in a clear stream flicking my line with a magic fly and reeling in a fighting fish, glistening silver through a streaming rain. Though once I did catch a Coho salmon with a rod and reel, when a dear friend at Schooner Cove thought I should have this experience.

Will I, as the late Queen Mother did with Diana, ever advise a grandson's prospective bride how difficult it would be to marry into my family? That is a possibility, and I can hardly wait. I've already changed my place of residence — not because I had to give it over to a daughter like the Queen did, but I have had to give up a second home to a son and his family.

I wonder if Queen Elizabeth felt as I did when she left Buckingham Palace for Clarence House? Oh I know, she wouldn't have pangs at seeing a familiar breadboard now being used without its former leather hanging thong, or the brown vase on the mantelpiece that always held seasonal day lilies or iris, or the special matching pillowcases, sheets and curtains in the bedrooms. Nor would she miss a real birch bark canoe, covered with winter dust, hanging above crowded bookcases. Nor a bathtub and bidet she was used to, nor even the smell of Buckingham Palace's family entry, the muffled sounds of crowds outside. At the particular sound of the click of her bedroom door after her lady-in-waiting had said, "Goodnight Ma'am," she could settle into what had been one of her own beds for how many more years.

Did she still miss her husband?

> *After hearing two eyewitness accounts of an auto accident,*
> *it makes you wonder about history.* — Anonymous

Buttermilk

she told him
shake harder
faster
faster

golden globules floated
the grandmother
buttered bread
smacked buttermilk lips
held the glass to the child
who grimaced
took his taste buds
to his computer

A Woman Who Cooks,
Eats, and Talks About It

At eighty-four-years of age, I'm not in the generation of women who run marathons or bungee-jump, and I eat sensibly. I do watch over two daughters and two daughters-in-law and seventeen grandchildren, ten of whom are female. We all eat, but differently.

One daughter cooked for her family mostly as she remembered I did when she was one of our five growing children. She observed me cooking for our ranch-hands. Later, she was one of my kitchen-helpers when I pulled out all the stops and became Martha-like though this was before Martha became Martha. We had large parties of seventy-five people held on consecutive nights in our home in the city of Edmonton, where I served buffet menus such as:

Mostly Wild Charcuterie:

- terrine, elk, bear and duck pâtés
- Rabbit compote
- Grape leaves stuffed with rice and elk
- High-country pâté
- Elk and moose sausage
- Romaine and elk strips with nasturtium vinegar and basil oil
- Pesto pasta

- Ratatouille, wild mushrooms with lemon and parsley
- Fennel olives
- Homemade mayonnaise with basil
- Lime mustard
- Sweet-and-sour pepper jelly
- Apricot chutney
- Pickled peppers,
- Cherries with gin and juniper
- Homemade herb bread
- Foccacia, onion and walnut breads, chocolate pâté and wheatmeal biscuits
- Lemon curd and shortbread, grapes
- Stilton and walnut torta and water wafers

Country Fare:

- Elk pâté
- City cousin pâté, pork loin with pear mustard, Plain Jane turkey roasted with wild plum and basil jelly
- Tiny wild rice pancakes with red pepper jelly with homemade herb and onion breads, rye bread with juniper butter
- Phyllos filled with onion and apple purée or cheese and apricot chutney
- Stuffed grape-vine leaves, smoked trout rillettes with marigold petals
- Salad bar Banked vegetables — some raw, some steamed and different dips — tapanade, quark cheese with red pepper anchovy relish, quark with basil pesto and cottage cheese, dill and yogurt
- World's largest pecan pies (cooked in paella pans)
- Apple tarts Lemon curd for shortbread old cheddar and grapes

This same daughter, Jody, gave her children: meatloaf, hamburgers, bacon and pancakes, roast beef, spaghetti and meatballs, roast chicken, mashed potatoes, and salad with iceberg lettuce mixed with baby greens. They used ketchup on real macaroni and cheese and she made minestrone soup, ginger and soft sour-cream-raisin cookies. She bottled five kinds of fruit chutney and made Christmas fruitcakes for me and her sister, as well as fudge and always homemade-to-measure birthday cakes. Her "pie-a-month- for-a year" donation was a popular neighborhood fundraiser. And she still makes a wonderful butter chicken.

My daughter Lori, restricted with multiple sclerosis, grilled tofu slices with hoison sauce. Her children snacked on fruit leather, cut up apples and oatmeal cookies, and she bought good bread.

I still can't help myself. In season I buy cases of preserving jars, soak labels off old jars for recycling, and beg jars from friends. Then I'm back in a steamy kitchen, tiny as the first kitchen I cooked in sixty-four years ago. For the last number of years, my production has shrunk since I only occasionally sell my wares — only preserves for gifts. Lately, my shelves and freezer have held: pickled cherries with gin and juniper, pickled plums, crooked asparagus relish (because I buy less-expensive, just-picked but crooked asparagus), sweet and sour pepper jelly, lime marmalade with shredded zucchini, tomato jam with orange and Worcestershire sauce (great on toasted tomato or chicken sandwiches, or stirred into pasta), lemon balm vinegar and yellow tomato ketchup.

For my freezer I make lemon and lime curd, jars and jars of it, to go on ginger cookies purchased from the Ikea furniture store. Also from Ikea are the round-lidded boxes I be-ribbon and fill with white chocolate bark, which calls for pistachios and dried cranberries, but I use toasted almonds or whole hazelnuts. I add to the dried cranberries scissor-cut crystallized ginger, dried apricots and mango. I also make and box addictive pumpkin-seed brittle with cumin. I store these boxes in my fridge alongside the paperwhite narcissus bulbs, whose roots twine amongst glass marbles, waiting to be brought one by one into room temperature and light. Then they will come into fragrant bloom on my kitchen table before Christmas.

Mini pound cakes with added lemon balm or lemon thyme sit in companionable rows in my fridge's freezer door. Sliced while frozen, these morsels thaw before I can get them on the side of a teacup. They share space with same-sized banana-coconut loaves studded with preserved ginger, apricots, and brazil nuts.

My harvested lemon thyme and lemon balm and mint in brown paper bags have long-since been taken down from their hooks on my kitchen ceiling. Their dried leaves rest in jars on my herb and spice shelves. I've thought of, once a month, removing all the lids for a few hours, and letting the smells mingle and waft through the house, but decided against such extravagance.

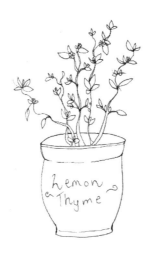

You wouldn't think that at eighty-four I'd still be buying cookbooks, but I am. I used to subscribe to *Martha Stewart Living*. Then a friend from England brought me the first of Nigella Lawson's cookbooks, and I've bought the rest. I watch her on TV and have sent away for sheet gelatin and paste colors, which I've tried only twice, but give me time, give me time. That Nigella. She makes Martha seem even more plodding, though Nigella does appear to have limes, mint, tumeric, cumin, coriander and feta cheese in seventy-five percent of her dishes. Why doesn't she pass her hands through running water more frequently, because she does lick her fingers often. And she makes dishes in which eggs aren't cooked and we're warned that this is currently a no-no though she gets her fresh eggs from Italy and maybe there's an Italian hex on botulism. To read about her love life in Vanity Fair adds to my interest in this voluptuous kitchen goddess.

My latest favorite TV chef is a Canadian: Laura Calder. She has three cookbooks: *French Food at Home, French Taste*, and *Dinner Chez Moi*. She has simple themes on her program, washes her hands when appropriate, and everything she does with droll humor makes sense.

I've very recently come to know Judith Jones' food writing. She edited Julia Child's famous books, among others, and has published her own book, *The Pleasures of Eating Alone*. Her ideas about food also show great common sense. Her book gives many variations on foods and her "second and third rounds" are what I've always known as leftovers. Her improvising ways are my tweaking ways and I *always* understand her motives. Some of Judith's "second-round" ideas are ones I'd never thought of and could very well be "first-round" candidates.

She talks about beef and kidney pie. This reminds me of the steak and kidney pie I made for Hu's birthday for many years. Not one of our children liked the small chunks of kidney in the filling, but their dad loved the whole thing and smiled all through dinner.

And I admire Jamie Oliver's frantic but courageous quest to change England's and then America's eating habits. Wonder if it works, will he try it in Canada?

I got into a bit of trouble with some members of my family who thought me terribly extravagant when I sent for a tiny pill-bottle sized order of edible gold flakes. These were for gourmet dinner desserts, and to be sprinkled on Xmas cookies to amaze grandchildren. If I live to be a hundred, I will still have some of this lovely light recklessness, since a little goes a very long way.

Are you wondering what a single older woman of today eats? Probably not, but I'm going to tell you anyway. Here are sample dinner menus for the past week when, except for Sunday, I've been at home alone. This is an average week, though I do on occasion get on a kick when I can eat the same dinner twice in a row.

- Monday — Leftover cold roast beef, baked potato with no-fat yogurt and real butter, and chopped green onion, sweet and sour pepper jelly. Green salad with dried cranberries. No dessert.
- Tuesday — Chicken stir-fry with fresh ginger, onions, green pepper, carrots, broccoli, half basmati rice and half brown, with low sodium soya sauce, half a banana with no-fat yogurt, honey and toasted almonds.
- Wednesday — Liver and onions, jasmine rice, sliced tomato, raw carrots, tomato jam, baked pear with yogurt, thawed angel food cake (When I bought the liver, a young man in front of me at the grocery store line-up said, "Ugh — liver. How can you?" and I replied, "It's good for you and I'm eighty-four." He: "How often do you have it?" Me: "Oh, maybe once a year.")

- Thursday — Curried, creamed canned-salmon and peas on toasted home-made poppy-seed bread, thawed mixed raspberries, blueberries and blackberries with honey and yogurt and 2 brownies.
- Friday — Bought "Lean Cuisine," green salad, a mandarin orange and 2 brownies.
- Saturday — Small, hot baked sweet potato on top of a cold mixed green salad, ice cream with maple syrup and toasted almonds.
- Sunday — Spring rolls with chutney tahini sauce, roast pork, glazed potatoes, carrots with dill, yogurt with cucumber, basil and sunflower seeds. Warm plum torte with ice cream (some of my children and grandchildren were here.)

When I have guests for lunch, I nearly always have soup. In the summer, it's cold — a watermelon or vegetable gazpacho, or fresh pea soup. Autumn brings a squash or similar bisque, and in winter I serve chicken-with-a-twist soups. I have a variety of fresh cheeses, always some chevre with, either my own bread, or good purchased loaves, my sweet and sour pepper jelly and tomato jam, and a fruit torte for dessert. I like a plum torte with pine nuts or pear with almonds and drips of Poire William. These both freeze well. I make two at a time and freeze one. Reheat a frozen torte in the microwave and it'll be as though you've lifted it freshly baked from your oven. Then sieve over with powdered sugar.

After all these years, I'm still a woman who loves to eat, cook and talk about it. In fact, I find it hard to stop, so here's the detailed story of a chicken stir-fry:

My neighbor's mock orange branches are nicely inching their way onto my side of the rough brown fence and it's blossom time. I've set the small, round, white cast-iron table with a blue-and-white fringed cloth. My dishes are the kitchen ones, Royal Doulton, blue and white with grapes and leaves.

Tonight it's a quick stir-fry. No need to use the rice cooker, since there's a small bag of leftover rice in the freezer. I put it in a bowl in the microwave to turn on later. From my windowsill I take two cloves of garlic from a shedding half-bulb. From my fridge's vegetable crisper I take one small leek, two carrots, two stalks of celery, a third of a red pepper, a frond of bok choy, a small handful of snow peas, and eight musky mushrooms from a softly wilted brown paper bag. From the shelf above, a chunk of ginger root, a jar of toasted sesame seeds and a bottle of light soya sauce. From the fridge freezer I take one small boneless chicken breast. From the cupboard next to the fridge I lift out the box of cornstarch and bottle of grapeseed oil. From the blue basket on the shelf under the kitchen counter I take the last very small onion, nestled like the last egg in the straw of a henhouse.

I cut the frozen satin-smooth chicken into thin strips, then dredge the pieces in cornstarch. Its smooth crunchiness makes a paste, which sticks to the chicken and to my fingers. I wash my hands and chop the ginger, licking the pungent remnants off my fingers, then wash my hands again. Then I chop the garlic but I do not wash away that permeating Italian, Chinese, French smell. Next, I cut three inches off the green end of the leek, and a thin slice off the base of the bulging string-rooted white bulb and push these parts into the garburator. The leek tops spin around in a whirling dervish dance until they disappear. I slice the leek lengthwise, rinse away the sand, and cut cross-wise pieces. I peel the carrots into the sink, then cut them into slanted chunks, one of which I eat with a satisfying crunch. I cut the bottom off the celery and string it into the sink. What's left is cut into crisp green arched pieces, some of which I eat with more crunches. I seed the red pepper and slice it into curved, crisp red strips, some of which I eat with less noise. Next I cut the bottom off the base of the bok choy, trim the green tops and slice crosswise. Then the mushrooms are cleaned, partially stemmed and sliced, some of which I eat. I slice the onion into thin rings. The garburator apologetically chews what should be in a compost pit but because I don't have a real yard, I can't be a proper environmentalist. I put the tea kettle on to boil for green tea.

I glug oil into the wok, and turn the burner to medium-high. I toss in the ginger and garlic. In a flash, my kitchen smells right. I'm careful not to burn the garlic and ginger, and remove them after a few minutes. I turn up the heat to high. The oil is now flavoured, so in goes the chicken. With tongs I turn these pieces. When pressed, they become more solid. With a spatula I toss the leek and onion, next the mushrooms. I stand tossing and turning these ingredients while the steam from them rises, curling my hair with a Chinese restaurant smell. Next carrots, celery, bok choy — toss. They become glossy. The leek tops and bok choy leaf shreds become a dazzling green and the onion rings are almost limp. I turn on the microwave two minutes for the rice. To the wok I add red pepper and snow peas, the garlic and ginger — toss. The pepper strips are the color of ultra-red lipstick and the snow peas glisten like grass after a spring rain. I sprinkle soya, and the brown and black speckles of sesame seeds — toss. Then remove the wok from the heat. Next, spoon the rice onto a warm waiting plate, add soya, and dribble the wok mixture over it. I go outside with a tray loaded with this plus a teapot of green tea, cup and saucer, knife and fork, no chopsticks.

I sit alone but am content. Next to my fence is a sidewalk where students trudge home from university. Seated, I can't see them but I hear their laughter and quiet chatter. I wonder if they're going home to wok dinners or if some are facing solitude and will be holding a book in front of a plate of Kraft dinner, or a re-heated slice of Funky Pickle pizza left over from the night before.

What I should do sometime is hang over my fence, watch for an undernourished looking specimen, and invite him or her to join me. I always have leftovers that I use the next day mixed with chicken broth. I could make an exception, but not tonight.

> *'Tis an ill cook who cannot lick his own*
> *fingers.* — William Shakespeare

Some of the Recipes:

Sweet and Sour Pepper Jelly

- 2 c. finely chopped red, and other colored seeded peppers
- ¼ c. or less, seeded jalapeno peppers (or leave out)
- 1&1/2 c. white or cider vinegar
- 1 tsp. salt
- 6 & 1/2 c. sugar
- 1 box (2 pkg.) liquid fruit pectin

1. In two or more batches, chop peppers to fine texture in food processor, using some of vinegar as liquid.

2. Put in large kettle with remaining vinegar and salt..

3. Place over medium heat, bring to boil, lower heat, simmer.

4. Stir occasionally five minutes. Stir in sugar.

5. Bring mixture to a full rolling boil (can't be stirred down) over high heat, stirring constantly, and boil for 1 minute. Remove from heat.

6. Stir in pectin. Mix well.

7. Skim off foam with metal spoon.

8. Stir and skim for at least 5 min. to cool slightly to prevent floating fruit.

9. Ladle into hot sterilized jars, filling to within ¼ inch of rim.

10. Process jars in water bath 10 minutes.

Spiced Tomato Jam

- 2&1/2 c. prepared tomatoes
- 1 peeled, sectioned and chopped med. Orange
- 1 tbsp. Worcestershire sauce
- ¼ c. lemon juice
- 1&1/2 tsp. lemon rind
- ½ tsp. ground cinnamon
- 1 box fruit pectin crystals
- 4&1/2 c. sugar

1. Scald, peel and chop tomatoes.

2. Place in large saucepan; bring to boil, simmer 10 minutes, stir.

3. Add chopped orange, Worcestershire sauce, lemon juice, rind and cinnamon.

4. Stir fruit pectin crystals into spiced tomato mixture.

5. Put saucepan over high heat. Stir till mixture comes to full boil.

6. Stir in sugar.

7. Continue to cook and stir over high heat until it reaches a full rolling boil.

8. Boil hard 1 minute, stirring constantly.

9. Remove from heat.

10. Stir and skim foam for 5 minutes to prevent floating fruit.

11. Pour quickly into hot sterilized jars filling ¼ inch from rim.

12. Seal while hot with sterilized 2-piece lids with new centers.

13. Process 10 minutes.

Plum or Pear Torte

For 2 9" spring-form pans. Each serves 8-10.

- 2 c. sugar
- 1 c. butter
- 4 lightly beaten eggs
- 2 c. flour
- 1 tsp baking powder
- abt. 16 halved prune plums or 2 pears sliced in 8's
- 4 tbsp sugar
- 2 tsp cinnamon
- 4 tbsp. Lemon juice and rind of one lemon

To sprinkle: pine nuts or almonds & splats of Poire William

1. Preheat oven to 350, butter and flour pans.
2. Cream together sugar with butter.
3. Add lightly beaten eggs, then flour and baking powder.
4. Beat, then spoon into pan.
5. Place cut side down on batter, abt. 16 halved prune plums or 2 pears sliced in 8, all mixed with sugar, cinnamon, lemon juice and rind of one lemon.
6. On plums, sprinkle pine nuts. On pears- almonds & splats of Poire William.
7. Bake 1 hour.
8. These tortes freeze beautifully but be sure to wrap them well in foil.

Pumpkin Seed Brittle with Cumin

- 1 ½ c. sugar
- ¼ c. light corn syrup
- 2 tbsp. butter
- ¼ c. water
- 1 tsp. sea salt
- ¼ tsp. baking soda

- 1 tsp. cumin
- 1 ½ c. green pumpkin seeds

1. Mix sugar, corn syrup, butter and water in saucepan and cook over med. heat. No stirring till caramelized -abt. 15 minutes but watch carefully. Don't burn.

2. Remove from heat, stir in salt, baking soda, cumin. It will bubble and froth. Add seeds and stir.

3. On a buttered baking sheet with a wooden spoon, spread mixture and score with a knife in long rows. When brittle cools, break it into shards.

My Scarf Drawer

On top of the mahogany chest of drawers sits a fax-copier-printer, piles of computer paper and photos. One would suppose the dresser's first drawer would hold more writing supplies but no, it contains panties, bras, and eighty antique handkerchiefs given to me on my eightieth birthday by daughter Lori. (Elderly women's noses drip and then there are all those funerals.)

The middle drawer holds knitwear; the bottom drawer: scarves. I sit on the carpet, pull open the scarf drawer, rummage and lift each delicate sample. Memories meander in my mind. My scarves remind me of people, places, events, sounds, smells, smiles and tears.

This long black and white streaked Italian scarf was my mother's. She wore it with a mink-trimmed black suit at my father's funeral. The suit was new and I remember my mother's drawn face when she said, "Bruce always liked me to look nice." In her way, she was honoring him, and in her understated way, was remembering. Remembering a marriage of forty-five years beginning at the time of flappers and prohibition before the stock market crashed. She met him at a tea dance at the MacDonald Hotel where they may have danced the Charleston though they never taught me how.

This silk chiffon length of mottled grey, yellow and leaf-green, fine and light as a yellow emperor moth's wings, could slip easily through my mother's engagement ring. The ring I gave my son Jeff to give his bride-to-be when they were both poor and in medical school.

These cotton scarves, partly spotted, white and blue, white and green, white and mustard, were neckerchiefs worn by Hu when he was riding his horse, Twister. My husband wore the white and blue one on his last ride. The day he died in the saddle, and I was there.

The formerly-white but now discolored-to-buff length of crepe was at the neck of my first maternity suit — grass green, as I was, with a hole in the front of the skirt, for the ballooning stomach to hide under the tent-like top. We bought it in October 1948, when Hu was doing some work at the University of Chicago. We were both so excited because I was one month pregnant with our first child. I wore the suit on the train, but didn't tell the customs official that I had purchased anything.

The white with pale hyacinth squares and hyacinth rolled-hem scarf went with a matching suit Hu bought me after Lori, our fourth child, was born. It was April. I thought of yellow and mauve Easter jellybeans. A faded picture shows me in this suit, the natural curl out of my hair due to birthing anesthetic, holding a swaddled infant.

My mother took better care of her good possessions than I ever did. Now I think I am more careful than my daughters were. My daughters' scarves poured crumpled out of their young daughters' costume boxes, scarves worn by their mother, grandmother and great grandmother. Cashmere and silk neckerchiefs, woolen shawls, silk oblongs and squares, navy, red and camel, green, orange and black, blue, yellow and pink, Indian, Italian, American, Liberty of London, French designer, silk-knit, striped, dotted, paisley, plaid, hand-painted, long and short, mixed with tulle tutus, hats with feathers, hand-made scarves by Simone from my bridal trousseau, a satin and lace nightie with matching peignoir. I don't know what ever happened to those wide-legged matching panties with their lace inserts and one pearl button on the side, fastened with a satin loop. They probably fell apart after too much bleaching from the days when blood streaks were a part of my life.

And this one, a silk square of peach and grey with a fantasy bird has been worn so often its off-white silk lining shows wear-lines, its "Maggie Rouff — Paris" signature is fading. I bought it in England for my mother. She shed to wear it swirled around her neck with a banker's grey suit. Is there still a faint smell of her Elizabeth Arden Blue Grass eau de cologne? I remember I wore it with a leather zip-up-the-front dress. In 1987 the Inter-Parliamentary Committee (American congressmen and senators with wives) joined their Canadian counterparts and we brought everyone from Ottawa to Banff and Jasper. A group picture shows me with Hu squinting at the camera next to our companions, me wearing this outfit along with a white wool jacket embroidered in peach and black that Hu brought me from his first World Bank job in Pakistan. This jacket sits in tiny splendor in the same cupboard where my wedding dress lies in a large box waiting for a maybe a granddaughter's wedding. Its ice-green satin and ecru lace has been remodeled once for Jody's first marriage (by my friend Simone who'd made my wedding lingerie and was back in town). Didn't bring Jody the luck it gave me. Lori didn't want any part of it when she married after her dad died. Her wedding was performed by a Justice of the Peace in our living room.

These two lengths of orange and blue silk chiffon were on a tweed turban I made to go with a matching Chanel-style suit. I remember patient little Danny playing with his Dinky Toy trucks on Madam Ira's, my designer's, glass coffee table, while I had my numerous fittings. I used to be thin. Never weighed over 118 pounds and wore a 32A bra that was padded with Kleenex.

This sky-blue large silk square, with its tiny dark-red rolled hem has four large, tangled masses of luscious fat raspberries with moss green leaves. Mother wore this under a black suit but I wear it with a red sweater and jeans.

The wide-bordered green square with its inner pattern of funky paisley in shades of grey, pale green and red always went with a stylish, rough collared-green tweed winter coat. In those properly-hatted days, I wore a small round black felt, the size of a bread and butter plate, with feathers that could have been from a crow. They stuck backwards out of a velvet rosette. The coat was warm, flecked with black and fastened comfortably high at the neck. I wish I had it now, but skip the hat.

I keep this ugly emerald green nylon georgette large square for memory's sake only. When I was modeling, we all had such scarves to place over our 1950's, heavily sprayed, puffed-up hair-do's. It went over our faces and tied quickly under the chin. It kept our stiff hair perfect and our makeup off the expensive designer outfits the dressers would drop over our heads.

This red-bordered, stylized Liberty of London silk paisley in white, red, green and yellow was my Christmas scarf. For how many years did I wear it on Christmas Eve, on Christmas morning and at dinner along with a long zip-front, dark green wool jersey hostess dress? I wish I still had that dress, though now it would be too tight. Oh, those Christmases — Hu, Tommy, Bruce, Jody, Lori, Jeffrey, Danny, Mother, Dad, Muriel and the rest. I smell white hyacinths, baby powder, roasting turkey, the open fire with mandarin orange peels and saved Nabob coffee packages, which perfumed and colored the flames. I hear our children singing "Silent Night."

This very large square scarf, its white jacquard background with every other colour including a small smattering of metallic gold, is a paisley that goes over a shoulder and hangs down front and back. This gives some lightness to an otherwise basic black turtleneck and pants. This way of wearing a scarf was dreamed up on an Italian fashion runway to sell even more expensive, large silk squares, which could be framed and hung as pictures. Not mine.

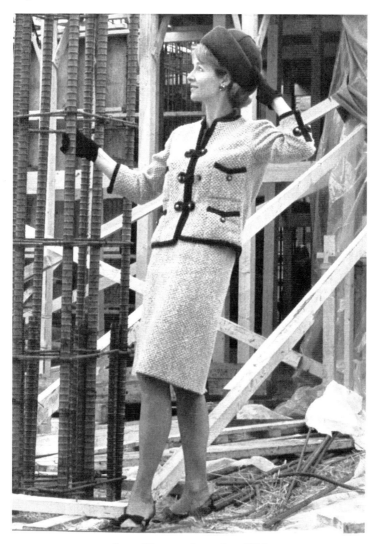

Joyce Edmonton Journal — 1954

As I look at these three long bias cut Liberty of London lengths of silk, orange-red, with pink, lime, turquoise and safflower angled stripes, intermingling with red and white small checks, and two blue-shaded beauties, I realize I haven't used them for at least ten years. Nor have I worn for ages these eight Sylvie Bouchard of Montreal three-inch-wide doubled silk lengths of hand-tinted art in ages. I bought them over a three-year period at craft fairs. Their subtle color combinations went with everything I owned and I used to wear them circled once around the neck and looped in front. The fickleness of fashion. Though there are basics in scarf styles, there are also trends. The Queen still wears a practical headscarf in the country, as did Audrey Hepburn and Bridget Bardot too, when their hair poofed-up high. Now, women let their hair blow, or if need be, pull a crunchable hat down over their ears and low on their foreheads. Scarves are for tying around necks, or substituting for belts in jeans. Frayed antique lengths get wound around and around long young necks. Old necks need camouflaging so I'll keep my collection for just that purpose.

Here's a scarf I seem drawn to. Teenage granddaughter Tasli wants me to will it to her. Time and time again, I twine its loopy length of pink, red, brown, black, purple and cream around my neck. It goes with everything except green or yellow.

There are many more soft, folded scarves in this bottom drawer. The scented tissue they sleep on beside their friends is old and wrinkled, just as they are and I am, but where they have been are the places I have been. The words they have heard are the words I have heard. The people they have known are the people of my life.

Women and elephants rarely forget. — Dorothy Parker

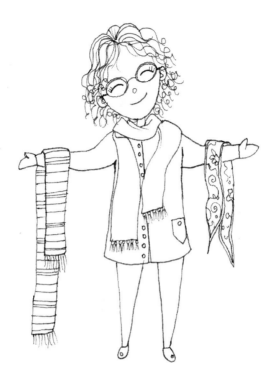

An American Girl in Italy

I looked at the large, now famous photo, in the Globe and Mail paper taken in 1951, and read the copy under it. It made me think: sixty years ago she was twenty-three, and so was I. While she was striding down a street in Florence, Italy, I was washing diapers and adoring my husband in Edmonton, Canada.

In the picture, Jinx Allen strides confidently down a hot morning street in Florence, Italy. Fifteen men of various ages ogle her. Two are on a Vespa, another one clutches his crotch, his mouth puckers in either a whistle or rude comment. I can't tell which, though today, the subject, much-married Jinx, insists this was an automatic gesture made for luck, not directed at her — just a guy thing. Not directed at her? Come on Jinx, but of course it was.

The photographer, Ruth Orkin, had her model repeat the walk and the picture was snapped. Perhaps some of these unemployed Italian men, hanging around five years after the war, are eying only the photographer, so I wonder too what she looked like.

Detective-like, I question published facts of a hot day, since Jinx is wearing a shawl and the men wear jackets or sweaters. And why are Jinx's eyes closed? Avoidance of the facts or just a fast photographer's shutter?

What is really true, beside the world of diapers and my lovely husband in Edmonton, Canada, 1951?

You are never too old to be what you might have been. — George Eliot (1819-1880)

Fiction

Kneading

She is glad their two girls are away at college, 'though she misses them desperately. They'd each spoken to her before they left.

Jeanine said, "Why do you stay with the old Grump?"

Angela pleaded, "Leave him Mom, you're too nice for him."

It is now two a.m. She'll make bread although it isn't bread-baking day. She dumps yeast into lukewarm sugared-water and puts two kinds of flour, white and multi-grain, in the extra-large mixing bowl. Looking at the yeast's gray bubbles she sighs and thinks, *that's my life — gray, gray, gray. But the worst of it is, I'm so lonely. Oh well, at least the freezer'll be full if I have a hospital stay.* She adds hot water, butter, honey and salt to the dry ingredients and then to the proofed yeast, till the mass is well blended. Then she kneads this large lump 'til, after about ten vigorous minutes, her practiced palms and fingers know it's time to rest the covered dough at the back of the stove. In between kneading, she pounds the dough as though it is her husband's thick chest.

Earlier, when she lay beside him in their old-fashioned double bed, she had been unable to tell him what she had known since last Tuesday. She'd been to the breast clinic where a mammogram showed a suspicious cloud. Not large, but as the doctor said, "A bit of a concern." Later this morning she must go to the hospital for more tests.

She and her husband had never talked much in bed or at the dinner table, or when they were working side-by-side heaving bales into the hay-barn or at the pens, knee-deep in gumbo. She remembered when they were courting and their early-married years. His energy and boy-like ways with their daughters grabbed her heart, though he never had been talkative. Now, his response to her comments or questions was often a piercing look, no answer, or else he would curse.

Her true nature was an upbeat one. How else could she have lived since 1980 with this man she married? She kept thinking, *He must still love me. He just can't show it any more. He's too full of anger: anger at Mad Cow disease, at stock prices, at Americans, at Japanese, at anyone in government. He gets furious at a slow driver in front of him, a dog barking in the night and he's angry with our daughters for going to college and leaving us with all the farm work. He's angry at the whole world, including me. What have I done? He's wound up tight as the spring on the screen door out back.*

She gives up the thought of any more sleep, and eases out of her side of the bed, pushes her feet into slippers and pads to the dark kitchen. She takes a heavy brown cardigan from a hook in the pantry, puts it on over her knee-length nightie, then a bibbed apron over that. She stares out the window at the barnyard. A strong wind makes the yard-light swing from side to side while it shines off and on the corrals, pump house, chicken coop and one end of the horse barn. A straggly pink geranium plant she'd held over winter on the drafty windowsill is almost ready to plant out. *Wonder if I'll get to do it or to plant the rest of my spring garden?* Last night at the dinner table, her husband had sworn, "We'll probably get at least one more god-damned blizzard and the god-damned cows'll calf and we'll lose some of the god-damned little buggers we don't need anyway," and he grabbed his pie plate, clunked it on the counter next to the sink, and pushed out the back door. Some days she ached from trying to see the bright side. When she did, he would sneer and swear at her chirpiness. There was little laughter in their home, although he seemed to be able to pull himself together in front of some of their close neighbors, sometimes even smiling at next-door neighbor Jim's lame jokes.

She pulls on green gumboots over bare feet and trudges to the hen house, surprises the birds by turning on the light, and finds three eggs. *Super-fresh for his breakfast, not that he'll thank me.* Returning to the kitchen, she sits in the chair at her end of the table, brings four gray work socks out of a bag and begins mending the heels. Ruefully, she thinks, *Wonder if he's cranky because his heels hurt. Nope, he's been like this since way before the Mad Cow crisis.* The kitchen wall-clock ticks away the time. The dough rises, pillowy and perfect. She gives it a whack, a mad satisfying whack, and plops it onto a large floured board. Dividing it in half, since her wrists can't handle such a large mass, she begins kneading and stretching, kneading and stretching, grunting as she works. She smiles to herself. *More cardio exercise and I don't have to go to a gym for it.* Presently, she gets the dough's correct elasticity. Grunting again, she completes both halves, divides them into twelve loaves, and plops them expertly into greased bread pans. She covers these with tea towels and glances at the clock. *Another hour or so before they go in the oven.* She checks the large freezer in the back larder. Just enough room left for eleven loaves of bread. (She'll save one for tonight). Already lodged in the freezer are bagged chickens, chicken soup, steaks, roasts, ground beef, beef stew, rhubarb, Saskatoon, and apple pies, crabapple juice, three sponge and three angel cakes. *Guess it's enough to keep him for a while.* She thinks more about telling him her news. *I hate always walking on eggs when I speak to him. Can't just come out and say, 'I'm to have more tests for a lump in my breast — hope things don't go the way they did for Grandma, Mom and Sis, 'else you'll be planting peonies at my grave too.' I can't get into his way of thinking. I can't.* She mulls over incidents of her husband's shows of anger and remembers, when once he'd said, "If I ever get cancer, I'll shoot myself."

The bread has risen beautifully, so she puts it in a moderate oven and sits idle, staring into space.

> *There is no such thing as pure pleasure; some*
> *anxiety always goes with it.* — Ovid

Tweaking

I call it *tweaking*, 'though others might not. They might call it changing a recipe. The difference being that, in my case, I never keep track. Those who change recipes mark in their cookbooks' margins such instructions as *substitute pine nuts for almonds, or 1/2 tsp. of cloves instead of 1 tsp.* or *needs 1/2 hr more in oven.*

My less structured way is to substitute as the mood strikes; perhaps some light coconut milk for part of the water in the rice pot. Toss some watermelon chunks in a salad on a hot day and crumble in some feta, Maldon salt and pistachios. Or, I taste, then stir more tart tamarind paste in the poached fish sauce, and paint chicken thighs with pomegranate molasses. I add lemon thyme to my grandmother's pound cake and extra Worcestershire sauce to my tomato marmalade. When making crooked asparagus relish, I save the tips whole, and mince the stalks in very small batches in the Cuisinart though the recipe says not to do this.

I remember my mother's look of distaste when my Aunt Maude proudly said she'd tossed stale cake pieces in the lunch custard. But I see the wisdom in this thrifty action. I've done it myself, but with plain yogurt. I added blueberries, crunchy apple slices, shredded lemon balm, toasted almonds and a trail of liquid honey over all.

I've never minded when a cold salad touched parts of a warm meal, so one day, an hour before I needed a nutritious lunch, I put a small sweet potato in the oven to bake. Next, I tore up some butter lettuce, sprinkled it with feta and dried cranberries and made a vinaigrette dressing. This last with three parts grapeseed oil and one part rice vinegar. Then in the bottle I pushed stalks of thyme and dill, dry mustard, sea salt, a bit of sugar, a splash of balsamic vinegar and a shake of Tabasco. I tossed the salad with the dressing, and dropped spoonfuls of hot sweet potato on top and tossed again. Hot over cold. It works.

When a banana-coconut loaf recipe calls for a cup of walnuts and maraschino cherries, I can use a larger quantity of a mixture — whatever I feel like — maybe chopped preserved ginger, dried apricots and/or cranberries, or raisins, and brazil nuts or almonds.

It's the freedom to keep to the basics, but add your own tweakiness that I'm comfortable with.

I watch food competitions on TV. A time-waster, I know, but I find my blood pressure rising as the clock runs down and the contestants show signs of last-minute meltdowns. I love how the secret ingredients the chefs deal with work their way into entrees and desserts never-before heard of. I hold my breath when contestants lift their monster many-tiered cakes to the judging table, sweat dripping from their hairlines. Not for me those programs of smart cops killing because they have to, or bodies with pen-marks on various areas where dermatologist surgeons will slice, dice and suture before ghoulish eyes. Nor do I watch the case-room dramas where families rejoice in the intensity of birth. And I haven't watched the shows that pit overly-fit young adventurers against one another. I don't need to see the ten most scenic kitchens in the world or what some of my least favorite food experts say about balanced diets. I already know about this topic. Nope, it's other kinds of food shows for me. They get my tweaking bones twitching.

If we keep on doin' what we've always done, we'll keep on gettin' what we always got. —Barbara Lyons

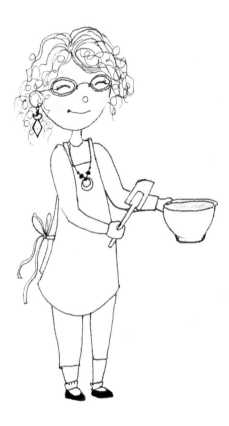

At a recent archaeological dig in England, it was found that legionnaires wore socks with their sandals.

So What

perhaps the only footwear they had
no cowboy boots brogues hip waders or reeboks
socks knit by each little missus back in Rome
needles clicked between
baby nursings and stomping grapes
when husbands abroad

why do we find it funny
seeing socks in sandals
we make it a sartorial crime

did this happen when Bridget Bardot
sauntered down a pebbled beach at St. Tropez
pouted at a hirsute male whose chunky
feet in Italian silk socks slid into sandals
said she preferred sun kissed men naked all over

Should One Eat Alone?

I read a headline the other day that, "He Who Eats Alone is Dead." If I stopped in at my local coffee shop in need of an orange walnut muffin (only to eat the crunchy topping, not the rather cakey middle and bottom) and a plain black coffee, would I pale, be turned into stone, a pariah, the object of pitying glances? I read the rest of the article, which quoted the writer, French philosopher Jean Boudrillard. He said that on his first visit to New York City he was shocked at a certain solitude like no other — the spectacle of adults eating meals all by themselves. He said, "It is the saddest sight in the world. Sadder than destitution. Sadder than the beggar is the man who eats alone in public. Nothing more contradicts the laws of man or beast, for animals always do each other the honor of sharing or disputing each other's food. He who eats alone is dead."

A bit of a stretch, old boy. How come Mavis Gallant talked about her joy when she first lived in Paris and saw a lone young woman in a restaurant eating oysters and drinking white wine while reading through a pile of newspapers? She even recalled the woman had a fruit tart for dessert. Gallant pointed out single women were not served in classy eateries in North America when she was in New York in 1950.

In my city, a single person is seated seemingly quite cheerfully at a table for two, and the extra place setting is removed from the tabletop with the server wondering what kind of tip a single will grace them with. Does this server wonder why I eat alone — often with a book? I've heard one shouldn't eat while reading, as the food will be eaten too fast, not relished with all one's senses. Maybe even encourage gastro-intestinal eruptions.

At home, alone of course, in front of the TV, dinner in a dim light, I glance at an interesting dinner-hour program, leaning over the plate to prevent dribbles, and I wish for a different scenario. Perhaps long narrow tables under an arbor in the Okanagan. August. Late August. No, late September when early ripening grapes are beginning to tempt birds, bears and deer. They too forage together. At the arbor's tables I will sit with the owner of this vineyard and some of his pickers. As is done in France, the hired help are fed generously at midday. Not enough to make them useless in the remaining hours to get the task done, but to revel in the remarkable crop. To talk about the perfection of conditions that produced such abundance. There is much laughter. So much laughter.

How could one bear to sit here and eat alone? And the food. It is hearty in a simple way. Cold, torn-apart roast chicken on platters. Big buns. Good big buns, in big baskets. Bowls of just-picked lettuce and tomatoes. Maldon salt in tiny bowls. Homemade mayonnaise. Pickled onions. Cheese boards. Slabs of lemon-and-chocolate cakes. Ripened pears. And wine — the house red and white, on the red and white checked tablecloths. What a dream.

What about a woman in hospital — propped against hard pillows, when the dinner table is rolled across her bed? On it, the tray of nourishment. Each dish chosen especially. Today, for her it is chicken soup. She can tell it's not made from free-range chickens. If she were to refrigerate it the mass would not jell. It is insipid — a noodled version of what she served her children when they came home from school for lunch on a cold February day. She dwells on her ailment, chews slowly, not savoring the fare. She thinks of past meals when she served a first meal to her new husband, all those family Sunday dinners and celebratory dinners marking family milestones.

Enough of this imagining. Jean Baudrillard, there is a place for solitary dining.

It's late April today and the forecast for tomorrow is light snow. Time to make my own solitary dinner.

*Seeing is deceiving. **It's eating that's believing**.* —James Thurber, *Further Fables for Our Time*, 1956

A Mickey of Gin

I need to buy a mickey of gin
you see
a friend swore
she took fifteen yellow raisins
soaked in gin
as a start to her day
and feels
her arthritis is disappearing
but I recall
hearing of crones in old London
and how they looked
from tippling gin
and wonder if they swilled it straight
or did the raisin recipe
reach back that far
though raisins
were soaked in sloe gin
by poachers
who dropped the fragrant doses
on trails through thickets
enticing animals
from their lairs on the lairds' lands
and did rabbits hop more freely
on their way to capture
and will my raisin regime
give more spring to my steps

Keeping Up

If ever I saw a startling face, it was the other night on TV when a clip of the late Helen Gurley Brown showed her talking to a young editor of her acquaintance. Helen was in her late eighties when this interview ran. She died recently at ninety. Her white teeth sparkled, her lips were dark red and fashionably puffed, her eyes twinkled though they were pulled tight, her voice was clear and lower pitched than it must have been when she was in her thirties — the era she appeared to be trying to copy. Her hair was dark and fluffy, showing no gray strands or pink old-lady scalp that I could see from where I sat in my TV room, nearly nodding off before tottering up to bed. She complimented the young woman who had taken her place as editor of *Cosmopolitan*, the magazine brought to prominence at the time of the second women's movement.

Helen's editorials and articles had shocked citizenry with their explicit sexual content. After all, in 1962 she wrote *Sex and the Single Girl*. It was during that period that she said, "Sex is one of the three best things out there, and I don't even know what the other two are." In 1982 when she wrote, *Having it All*, she occupied a significant role in the women's world, claiming she was an educator. I question whether much of the enlightenment has done us a whole lot of good. When I saw her, her skeletal hands gestured as she made her points and I thought of another woman of my acquaintance, not quite as old, who, at seventy, after birthing and raising seven children, (her husband died when the seventh was a baby), picked up and moved to a new country to be near many of her children and grandchildren. She suffers some serious health problems but sails on, her face telling her story, laugh lines and all. She makes new friends, young and old, rides her bike, takes university classes, influences her grandchildren. Her sphere is smaller, but, to me, seems more important than Helen's.

Then, another woman of my acquaintance, this one, at ninety-four, older than Helen, prefers the company of younger women. She says her friends are mostly dead and gone or "the old fools who are left dodder and one has to keep up." She does. She smiles and tells me she'd like a toy-boy to take her out for dinner occasionally or to a play, hold her arm so if she falls, they wouldn't both go down breaking all four hips. He would be able to see to drive at night. His digestive system would be able to handle scotch, pâtés and spicy foods, which she still can, although admittedly, in very small quantities–except the scotch, which she can still drink in moderation. She plays bridge, though a mixed poker game is more her style, and has taken to watching poker on TV, playing it at bedtime on her computer instead of solitaire.

She sides with her grandchildren and great-grandchildren, tells them how she felt as a teenager and young parent. Tells the girls what she has learned about men — how, "They are all little boys inside and one needs to treat them kindly."

Women of my acquaintance talk of the near future, when they will move to a senior's residence. Some dread being boxed with the elderly, although that's what they themselves are. They will be forced at mealtimes to listen to talk of ailments, doctors, pills, the latest medications found to be harmful and taken off the market and "however will I manage without it?"

We become timid physically, although we tell ourselves it is only wise to hold on to stair railings, dread icy sidewalks and look for restaurants with carpeting to dull the clatter, allowing us to hear our friends across the table. To confuse us, tiny print, often in pale green and translated from Chinese by Chinese whose English is far from perfect, appears on instruction bulletins with new gadgets or some pills.

Is it because there are more of us around that some youth don't treat us with the respect we were taught to deliver to the elderly? Or is it because the young have seen some of us as cantankerous old folks, shaking our canes at their fast-moving thoughtlessness, shouting our displeasure with forceful non-swear words they barely understand. The tone is explicit, but there is no eff-word in our string of expletives.

We need a reason to get out of bed in the morning. We wake up bright as a button, able to do anything if we have it marked on our calendar. Then, after lunch, we need a nap.

Sadly, there are some of us who are trapped. Unable to get out of the apartment to shop. The store is no longer on the corner. The library is too far away, two bus changes and anyhow, eyesight or attention-span doesn't permit reading for any length of time, or perhaps the habit was never developed. Bodies slump in front of the TV. Meals consist of tea and toast.

There's a limit to staying young. We are old and getting more-so every minute. We're told to not try to think about anything further ahead than two years. That sounds sensible though someone else says, "Take no long views, not much beyond dinner time." But the more I think about it, the more I want to stop and think about it tomorrow.

The trouble with life is that there's no back-ground music. — Anonymous

Sylvia Said

Sylvia Plath said
you can't talk poetically
about toothbrushes

of course many things upset Sylvia
including her husband
she thought he brushed her off
it now appears he had a bum rap

had she lived
could she have waxed poetic about
other brushes

toilet brush
hair brush
brush next to a solid male body
brush a voodoo doll's hair
brush away a cobweb
    tears
    table crumbs
    leaves off patio chairs
    cat hairs off her black skirt
    dust from patent leather pumps
      venetian blinds
      books
brush memory from the mind
brush with death

Think of Your Grandmother Naked

Have you seen the bumper sticker, "Think of Your Grandmother Naked"? This got me thinking of medical students and how at first they might be appalled to see what aging can do to the female body. From firm to flaccid, elastic to inelastic, silver stretch marks now on sagging skin, breasts closer to waist level than armpits. Hands and feet gnarled with arthritis.

They have seen young, glistening, buffed bodies toiling up hills, gulping water and tossing the bottles back to cheering crowds. The male student may have a live-in girlfriend who puts on the coffee while wearing only a purple-and-red paisley thong, her breasts perky, tan lines faint reminders of their sailing holiday.

Movies, TV, videos all show our young people what bodies "should be like," but where are they told that the bodies they see in hospital gowns can tell them stories? Stories of hands: Knuckles enlarged and knobbed, perhaps from weaving a darning needle up and over, up and over on the heels of hand-knit socks. Or punch and pull, punch and pull the wool strips through burlap, completing a hooked-rug for the back hall. Or punch and punch and press and push, kneading the dough to be placed under a clean white tea-towel to rise and be lifted, puffed and jiggling, to the oven.

A woman's silver stretch marks sometimes come and never go. They are silver medals, though they should be gold medals for building babies. It was said that rubbing cocoa butter on swelling stomachs and hips could prevent these everlasting stripes, though skin specialists will tell the students that only some skin types will be afflicted.

And breasts, some now removed, scarred where once snuffling babies gorged and husbands laid hands and heads.

And stories of feet, once dancing, twirling, carrying a young woman to the man who holds her tight and who may become her lover and lifelong partner. Her toes, now crooked, not able to waltz or jitterbug.

And knees, bending freely to pick up toys, pull carrots, pick poppies, scrub the kitchen floor, race up stairs to the sound of a crying infant, bend and kneel beside a dying child, husband or parents.

And mouths, with lips now smaller than in the ripe days when they smiled at lovers and babies. Now cracked skin surrounds wry grins as she thinks of the beautiful foolishness of youth.

There is no cure for birth and death save to enjoy the interval. — George Santayana, 1952

Aging in an Ordinary Way

I'm aging in an ordinary way. Age hasn't hit me like a fish biting a hook — quick and unexpected. It has arrived silently, like dribbling ice cream on hot apple pie. I listen to friends' reportage of how the passage of time is affecting them and I begin to make a list. So far, so good.

There has been a bit of a loss in the acuity of both my nose and my tongue. While I'm still able to sniff a rumor, burning toast and that beautiful baby smell, I've not smelled danger in years. As for my tongue, it seems to talk as much as ever, clucking over friends' ailments, and not being bitten often enough where some grandchildren are concerned.

The only thing kinky about me has been my hair, but recently it was brought to my attention that a book I wrote may not be suitable as a text for junior high school students. The comment that it could be warped, lewd, suggestive or even masochistic floored me. This was due to the book's title, *Girdles and Other Harnesses I Have Known*, which came from an essay in the book about women's clothing from 1928, the year of my birth, to the era when pantyhose was available. I like to think of it as a wise and gentle collection of memoirs, fiction, essays on aging and food, and poems.

I had preserved an innocence in these matters until recent years. All media have spelled out in too much detail the slices of humanity that indulge in practices beyond my comprehension.

It's not that I can decipher many of the words to songs blasted from stages needing chains and pyrotechnics to hype audiences, many who surprisingly sing along with those noisy performers. I have seen portions of current songs in print and my fusty sensibilities prevent me from repeating any of the lyrics. Where oh where is delicacy, lightness, tenderness? And where oh where is love?

I'm uncomfortable with brief moments I've seen on TV and need to click to PBS or the CBC or go to bed with a good book.

We're told seniors will lose three quarters of their taste buds by the time they're eighty, so food in seniors' facilities will seem more bland than for the young kitchen staff licking their tasting fingers. Anorexia of aging hasn't hit me yet, though with tightening waistbands, perhaps I should try it.

And have you heard? There's a new kind of taste sensation. For all these years, I thought salty, sweet, sour and bitter were all my tongue had to contend with. I'm now informed there's a new taste quality called umami. We're told that MSG (mono-sodium glutamate) is umami to the highest degree. It enhances like salt and harmonizes with other flavors. I remember being told, years ago, that MSG was a dietary no-no, a poison almost. What's happening here? As well, we're told dried mushrooms have more umami than do fresh. I should make my aged drying up years more umami-like. Flavor enhanced, suppressing bitterness and harmonizing with other ages.

That other kind of taste, you know, taste buds in the brain. Do we lose those too? Here I speak of aging women, knowing not a whole lot about aging men as my husband died at sixty-four. Or do we lower our standards, going for comfort instead of for fashion? Our feet are more likely to be in house slippers or Reeboks, and never in Manolo Blahnik's ankle-twisting creations. I watch TV programs where badly dressed people purport to correct a young person's unfortunate choice of clothing. Occasionally, I can agree with their advice, but would love to have their own wardrobes under my scrutiny. When I see runway fashions from New York or abroad, I wonder sometimes where the tiny garments modeled will be worn, and how cold so much of that bare skin would be in my neck-of-the-woods.

Then those house renovating shows, with their no-dints-in-cushions, hardly any family photos, everything white or off-white. What's wrong with color? No crumbs on the breadboard, impossibly fresh flowers everywhere and sound must ricochet in those two-story front foyers. Surely that's taste of another kind.

As I age in my very own ordinary way, I admire and enjoy my children, grandchildren and friends. I cook healthy food, read, breathe fresh air deeply, befriend and counsel young students and write letters to the editor. Oh sure, there are lapses of memory, but so far nothing too alarming. Knees ache, but I don't need surgery, and no Metamucil — just an apple-a-day. There's no depression or need for pills to maintain a proper serotonin level. Ordinary, almost a bad word, maybe *bor-ing*. No ring to it. No bells or whistles. One tone, like from the hospital's bedside machine with no blipping and bleeping. A straight line, but that denotes death. A far cry from that. I'm aging in an ordinary way.

> *"You grow up the day you have the first real laugh at yourself."* — Ethel Barrymore

I Heard It

why did he say it
on Whyte Avenue
to his cell phone

I heard it
he said
    with you on my arm
was he proposing marriage
walking west past me
in that instant
it was all I heard
    with you on my arm
I turned and saw his
bulky back
striding away from me

instead of going east
to the mailbox
I'll go west to see
if he's on his way to her

I caught up
followed
till he turned into a high-rise
and I walked past

holding my letter
still guessing

I cook with wine. Sometimes I even add it to the food. —W.C.Fields

Gelatinous Gems

I love jelled foods. Always have. The pleasure of holding a dollop in my mouth, waiting for it to melt into its own flavor essence, is sensuous. It's comfort food. No effort. It slithers down the throat like liquid or mercury in a thermometer. That's why Jello, like cubes of colored glass, are on many patients' hospital trays. It's supposed to contribute to a patient's well-being, especially after tonsillectomies. Grieving people need comfort food. Gelatin concoctions slide down crying throats. Gelatin provides the illusion of body, while possessing no substance of its own.

The commonly used jelling product is powdered gelatin. It comes from the bones and skins of animals, and was first manufactured in Holland in 1681. Leaf gelatin is another form from the same source and looks like small sheets of crackling cellophane. Four of these sheets equal one package of powdered gelatin. Professional chefs generally use these leaves, which can be found in gourmet and bakery supply shops.

Pectin is another jelling compound that's found naturally in apples and citrus fruits. This can be purchased in liquid or powder form (with directions enclosed), for preserving purposes.

Agar (agar-agar or Japanese gelatin) is a vegetarian jelling compound, which comes from edible seaweed. Agar agar flakes can be substituted for other gelatin. Unlike common gelatin, agar will set at room temperature. It can be found in Japanese or health food stores and is pricier than the other gelatins.

There are two steps for working successfully with the more common kind of gelatin. First, soak it (powder and leaf forms) in cool liquid to soften. In the case of the powder, stir the soft mixture into the boiling liquid. With gelatin leaves, squish out cool liquid with your fingers (interesting feeling, which I like) and put the limp mass into the hot liquid and stir to completely dissolve the gelatin. While these mixtures cool, the proteins join to form webs, which hold the moisture. This is called a gel. If you don't follow the rules, you'll have a grainy, rubbery or unset concoction, which you'll be unable to fix.

One envelope of regular gelatin contains one tablespoon of gelatin and will gel two cups of liquid. One tablespoon of agar agar flakes will gel one cup of liquid.

If you're making chicken in lemon aspic you use less gelatin in the stock, since it contains the natural gelatin from chicken bones.

There's a wonderful surprise jelly found under a poached chicken after it's sat in the fridge overnight and the broth's vegetables and herbs have left a faint memory. Scrape off the fat layer and the quivery mass can be cut into small dice, mixed with chopped green onion, parsley, lemon zest and a splash of Tabasco sauce.

A stunning, strong-tasting savory can be made by boiling balsamic vinegar, reducing it somewhat, then adding agar agar flakes, pouring it into a shallow pan, chilling, then turning out on a board and cutting into small squares. These dark, shimmering cubes can sit next to a salad or meat dish. It's a taste revelation.

Picture a clear golden ring of gin and tonic jelly on a hot day. Nigella Lawson surrounds it with white currants, though suggests powdered-sugar-covered red currants would do as well.

To end a festive dinner how about jellied champagne in flutes, blue borage flowers unsinkable on the slippery surface, or individual chocolate Bavarian creams, sitting in puddles of raspberry sauce. Nothing like the grade seven home economics puckery lemon snow where we learned about gelatin.

Old-fashioned Christmas always had a cloudy tower of tomato aspic, quivering on milk glass on the white damask tablecloth. This sat next to the Christmas turkey and cranberry sauce. The concentrated tomato flavor coated our tongues like cool satin.

What about Martha's Christmas citrus terrine which I served a few years ago and none of my grandchildren liked. (I don't know what's wrong with their young taste buds). All the adults loved its orange and grapefruit sparkle set in greens with shreds of beets and coins of radish.

Then there is salmon mousse — hat classic, pale-pink-and-green-flecked fish-shaped loaf, resplendent on elegant buffet tables in upscale hotels, clubs, and old Hollywood movies. This was before these venues moved to sushi, Thai wraps, tiny lamb chops, and mascarpone cheese with pomegranate molasses on fennel boats.

In my early married years during the late Forties, and early Fifties, Jello ice cream pies were the rage. A good piecrust was filled with Jello that had been softened with hot water and then ice cream was stirred into it. Fruit was folded in and they were called parfait pies.

When my children were very young, Valentines Day meant red Jello for lunch with some cinnamon heart candies (too spicy for the very little ones). We had bright green Jello on St. Patrick's Day. Canned fruit cocktail was a new product and was a sometime addition to red or orange Jello. Pre-schoolers were allowed to make the Jello for dessert. I can still see them, wearing my too-long apron, and standing on a chair opposite me, stirring slowly, after being cautioned to, "Be careful dear, it's hot — Good job."

What would church suppers, summer family reunions or country weddings be like without those glistening jellied salads? Bright green encasing shredded carrots and celery or pale green with cottage cheese, mayonnaise and pineapple? I am told, though have no wish to know details, that not only whipped cream, but Jello can figure in some porn movies.

Now, some mornings, I set a jar of my homemade crabapple jelly on the table, then begin balancing its quivering crimson fragments on my whole wheat toast, and think, "What a way to start the day."

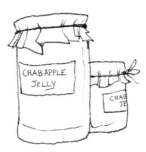

Some recipes:

Quick Tomato Aspic

8 servings

1. Soak 2 tbsp. gelatin in ½ c. cold V-eight juice.
2. Then dissolve this in 3 ½ c. hot juice.
3. Add dried basil and fine-chopped celery.
4. Mold, chill, unmold and serve.

Chicken in Lemon Aspic

Serves 8

Preheat oven to 350

- ½ c. oil
- 2 onions, sliced thin

- 3 celery stalks, sliced thin
- 4 large carrots, sliced thin
- 3 seeded lemons, sliced thin
- 6 to 8 garlic cloves
- Salt and pepper
- 3 to 4 lb. stewing chicken, cut into pieces
- 1 tsp. fennel seeds
- 4-oz. jar pimiento, sliced into strips, juice reserved
- ½ c. dry vermouth
- 1 c. white wine
- 2 tbsp. wine vinegar
- 1 to 1 ½ c. chicken stock (broth)
- ¼ lb. string beans
- 2 tbsp. gelatin

Heat oil in heavy casserole that can go in oven. Add sliced veg., slices of 1 lemon and garlic. Cover and simmer very slowly for abt. 20 min. until vegetables are quite limp but not browned. Sprinkle a little salt and pepper.

Remove two-thirds of veg., spreading the remainder evenly in bottom of the pot. Alternate chicken, veg., fennel seeds and lemon slices.

Mix vermouth, white wine, vinegar and pimiento juice and pour over chicken. Then pour on enough chicken stock to raise the level of the liquid so that it almost completely covers the ingredients.

Cover with a lid, and bake for abt. 2 hrs. Remove from oven, uncover and cool.

Place chicken pieces in colander over deep dish to gather liquid as it drips. Do the same with cooked veg. Combine this drained stock with the rest of the cooking stock. Cool and chill so the fat rises to the top and congeals; lift off the fat, and discard. Taste for saltiness. Remove meat from bones, discarding skin and bones. Separate meat into pieces.

Cook beans till tender. 5 or 6 min. Drain and cool at once under cold running water.

Soften gelatin in a little water, then heat it thoroughly in the stock until it dissolves. Cool.

Ladle thin layer of aspic into loaf pan mold, and chill to set. Put carrot slices in the middle and a red pimiento in center. Arrange string beans in spoke fashion, radiating from the carrots. Remaining string beans can be cut into short lengths and added to the cooked vegs. Carefully ladle in enough of the syrupy aspic, just to cover the veg. Chill until firm.

Put layers of chicken meat in the mold, alternating with layers of cooked vegs. Press very lightly with the palm of your hands, then pour in enough aspic to cover the ingredients. Chill for at least 1 day, 2 days is better. Extra aspic can be chilled to set, then chopped to decorate the platter.

At serving time, quickly dip mold in hot water and unmold onto serving platter. To slice, use a very sharp knife with a sawing motion.

Citrus Terrine

Serves 8-10

- 4-6 beets washed and trimmed, or 2 tins sliced beets, matchsticked
- 1 tsp. salt
- 12 oranges
- 4 pink grapefruit
- 1 c. fresh orange juice, strained
- 1 envelope unflavored gelatin
- Mixed salad greens
- 8 radishes, sliced paper thin
- Walnut Vinaigrette (recipe follows)

1. If using fresh beets, put in small saucepan and cover with cold water. Add salt and bring to boil over med. high heat. Simmer until tender when pierced with the tip of a knife. Drain and cool. Peel and cut into matchstick pieces. Do this to sliced, canned beets.

2. Using sharp knife, slice off stems and tips of citrus. Cut away peel and pith. Slide knife down one side of a segment, cutting it away from white membrane. Twist blade under section and lift out. Continue until all sections removed.

3. Pour 1/3 c. of the orange juice into a small bowl. Sprinkle gelatin evenly over surface and let soften10-15 min stirring once or twice. Heat remaining ½ c. juice to a simmer and combine with gelatin mixture. Stir well until gelatin has dissolved. Refrigerate until cool to the touch, abt. 30 min.

4. Line two 6-by-3 inch terrine molds with plastic wrap (loaf pans). Dribble a few tbsp of gelatin mixture in bottom of molds and arrange a layer of orange sections on this. Cover with more spoonfuls of gelatin, and top with layer of grapefruit sections going in opposite direction. Repeat until you've reached top of mold. Don't press down fruit. Fold plastic wrap over molds and refrigerate overnight.

5. When ready to serve, dip terrine molds into a bowl of hot water for a few seconds and invert onto a cutting board. Remove plastic wrap. Using serrated or very sharp knife, carefully cut into ¾ inch slices.

6. Arrange greens on each of the plates. Dress beets with some of the vinaigrette. Top greens with a slice of terrine and garnish with beets and radish slices. Drizzle salads with remaining vinaigrette

Walnut Vinaigrette

- 1 tsp balsamic vinegar
- 4 tsp fresh orange juice
- 4 tbsp walnut oil (or good olive oil)
- Salt and fresh ground pepper

Combine vinegar and orange juice in a jar and shake. Season to taste with salt and pepper.

Salmon Mousse

Yields about 6 cups
- Butter to grease mold
- 1 envelope unflavored gelatin
- 2/4 c cold water and ½ c boiling water, for gelatin
- ½ c mayonnaise
- 1 tbsp fresh lemon juice
- 1 tbsp fresh lime juice
- 1 tbsp grated onion
- 13 drops hot sauce
- ½ tsp paprika
- 1 tsp salt
- 2 c. poached or canned salmon, flaked into small pieces
- 2 tbsp capers drained
- 1 c. whipped cream
- Lemon slices
- Parsley
- Dill sauce
- 1 English cucumber, peeled, grated and drained for 12 hours
- 1 c. sour cream
- 1 c. mayonnaise
- 1 tbsp fresh lemon juice
- 1 small clove garlic, minced

- 1 tsp salt
- 2/3 c. fresh dill, finely chopped
- Grease a 6 c. fish mold or loaf pan with oil.

Soften the gelatin, in ¼ c. cold water. Add ½ c. boiling water and stir well till the gelatin has dissolved. Add mayo, lemon juice, lime juice, onion, hot sauce, paprika and salt and mix well. Fold in the salmon and capers. Add whipped cream and continue folding till everything is well combined.

Pour the mixture into prepared mold. Cover with plastic wrap and chill in fridge 8 hrs or overnight.

To make dill sauce: combine all ingredients in a med. bowl. Cover with plastic wrap and chill for at least 1 hour.

When ready to serve, unmold the mousse onto a platter. Take the lemon slices and create a "tail" on the back of the fish. Surround the mousse with parsley. Serve dill sauce in a glass bowl next to the salmon mousse

Panna Cotta

This Italian treat is an easy dessert that is smooth and light. It can be flavored with any herb, spice or liqueur.

- 4 c. milk
- 1 c. of any sugar
- 2 pkg. gelatin
- 2 tsp. pure vanilla
- 1 tsp. spice, herb or splash of liqueur

1. Pour almost all the milk into a small saucepan and gently warm over a medium heat. 2. Stir in the sugar, vanilla and any optional flavours. Continue heating until the mixture just begins to simmer.

3. Meanwhile, sprinkle the gelatin powder over the remaining milk. Let it rest for a minute or two as it begins to rehydrate

and absorb moisture. Pour in the hot milk and stir until completely dissolved.

4. Divide the mixture evenly between six small dessert moulds.

5. Refrigerate until firm, at least two hours or overnight.

6. To release the panna cotta, gently loosen the edges, cover with a small plate then flip over.

To eat is human; to digest, divine. — Mark Twain

A tribute to Al Purdy's Poem,
"At the Quinte Hotel"

Not at the Quinte Hotel

I'm drinking
I'm drinking tea with lime wedges
in my bedroom
on a hot summer night
you can see
….I'm a demure woman
there's a ruckus a raucous ruckus
under my bedroom window
it trolls down the street
as a young woman repeats
the eff word
….not a demure woman
….that's me
plugging one ear
and sipping tea
in the hot upstairs room
and though
…. I'm a demure woman
I don a raincoat over my
short summer nightie
and plunge outside
calling watch your tongue
what's wrong what's wrong

and the girl says the eff word
to me at me
my eighty-four-year-old sensibility turns cranky
I suggest calling the cops
the girl staggers
loses a flip-flop
spits the word
again and again
yells
I want to leave the effing party
so I say
can't you be more poetic
she sways says sure
mary had a little lamb
at least she didn't say
an effing little lamb
which would truly have bothered
my sensibilities even more

and I say
what about the perfume from
those lilacs
and she picks two
hands them to me
slurs sorry if we woke you
go back to bed

I put the blossoms
in a toothpaste glass
smell them round the corner
in the bedroom
don't say an effing good night
…'cause I'm a demure woman

Fiction

Dance to Discover

She was seventeen and hardly out of bobby socks and saddle shoes. She owned a red gabardine suit, which she wore with alternating white or grey blouses, and had a pair of gray sling-backed, open-toed high heel shoes, which she wore every day to work at an insurance office.

Then came the fire-engine salesman. At least that was what he was trying to be, and of course if he had, sold a fire engine that is, he'd have been in gravy for a year. In the meantime, he batched with his salesman brother.

She remembers once, at the brothers' apartment, on the ground floor of an unpainted old house in the middle of down-town, when the two young men had her help them in a task she supposed they didn't indulge in frequently. They were match-ing up tartan socks, knit by their mother, after they'd had a hand-washing marathon the night before. The trick was to put together matching pairs with no holes in the heels.

Her dad told her he wanted her to stop dating this young man. Juan *was* a bit racy looking for those late-Forties times — slicked back black hair and a black mustache. He wore pin-striped suits and rather loud ties. He holidayed in Cuba, had been discharged from the Canadian Air Force right after World War Two, and was an absolutely marvelous dancer. She was so naïve then. Didn't realize what the hard bump was at the front of his trousers when they danced close, which was most of the time. She didn't know the details of how things work. Fancy that, such innocence. Then too, he was of a different religion than her family, and her dad wanted to avoid problems on that front.

She met him under the ruse of going out with the girls — always necessitating secret phone calls and sleepovers with friends to back her up. She loved the excitement of it all. She got away with it, though fortunately for everyone, including Juan, she met another older man when she turned eighteen, whom her parents approved of and who was meant for her, so she lived happily ever after. Though every time she heard a fire engine's wail she wondered if Juan had sold it.

Funny though, years later, that same young man turned out to be a big oilman in Texas. She was told he and his wife had had three children under the age of one — twins and a single, and when she told her dad this, he said, "I never did like that fellow."

Dancing is discovery and recreation, especially...the dance of love.
Besides, it's the best way to get acquainted. — Leopold S. Senghor

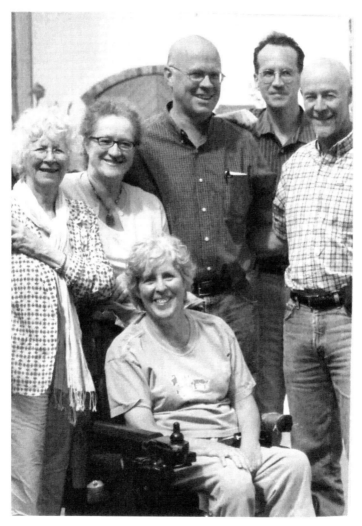

My 80th Birthday Party

Too Many Things

too many things
Christmas cake battered
crowded head
ingredients stuck together
children
grandchildren
problems
problems
she can't solve
if only
she could twirl
a spatula
around their lives
lifting problems
to splat
them over her right
shoulder
for luck

Now I Wish*

I tried, but with feeble efforts. Against my will, I was civil to her.

What made me be so cool toward my mother-in-law, Marian Osborne Harries? She was a woman I now know, after some years of mature reflection, who was surely undeserving of her only daughter-in-law's coolness.

To rationalize one's own bad behavior more than sixty years after the fact is difficult. And to come to some sort of semi-happy forgiveness of oneself is likely an exercise with which I shouldn't clutter my mind. Why bother? After all, I wasn't exactly the daughter-in-law from hell. And then, the passage of so many years will make from 1948 to 1952, while I knew her, seem either fainter or worse in my memory.

Did she think, *He adores her — she's so young — has eyes only for him — he'll treat her well — maybe she'll grow up and they'll have a wonderful life.*

And I, in my fluttering, immature mind might have been thinking, *She laughs in that tinkly way at things I don't think are funny and my ribs and stomach all go tight when she does it.*

I'm sure she was trying to lighten the tenseness about sharing her golden son with a young, inexperienced, unworldly woman. At the time I was too dense to know what was happening and my long-time regret is that I failed to become closer to her before her death.

And she kisses him if he's just going to the corner store. She looks so old. And she has so many ugly clay pots of plants on that table in the bay window. When I write these words today I shudder — so mean, so immature. What was wrong with me? There must have been something. Was I subconsciously jealous of Hu's obvious love for this strong but gentle woman?

Hu told me, "She always smelled natural gas," and at that aura sign, his mother would collapse, and he, a boy, though man-of-the-family, would put something in her mouth to keep her from biting her tongue, loosen her clothing, check to see if she'd maybe broken her leg, and wish his father were alive. Hu told me this, though I was never witness to his mother's epileptic seizures. When I was in the hospital with our first child, she had one, an episode in our tiny bathroom and he had to break down the door, hinges on the inside. I wondered at the paint chips on the pale blue and white wall though a first baby's cries changed the subject and we did not speak of it again until some years later, after Hu and his mother met with a committee of doctors deciding to sterilize his sister. Our children's only aunt. Muriel was ten-and-a-half months older than her brother and raised by their mother, a woman who had served overseas as a nursing sister in World War One and developed epilepsy afterward. She had scrimped and saved through the years after her husband's death, when Hu was fifteen, in order to provide for Muriel who would not then be a burden to her brother. Should my mother-in-law not be able to care for Muriel some day, she feared what could happen to her mentally challenged daughter. This daughter drank her tea like a lady, sat like a lady, rarely said a bad word, brushed her teeth morning and night and washed her hands after going to the bathroom. She was well brought-up though was not capable of looking after herself. And, she was fixated on having a family with little children like her brother had and was so gullible she could have been talked into anything even though she had been warned against men and their phony kindness. So the deed was done.

If I could do it again, I would ask Marian to tell me more of what it was like in the Peace River with those other four siblings, three of whom I met before their dotage, and all sounding and looking like they had stepped out of the top floor of *Upstairs, Downstairs* in Masterpiece Theatre. Marian herself looked and sounded like Dame Wendy Hiller. I was astonished one night, when flipping the TV channels, I came upon Marian, but it was Dame Wendy. There she was, white-haired, big smile, black dress, not a severe black suit like my mother- in- law usually wore, but there was a white lace jabot. Dame Wendy's skirt was long, so I couldn't tell if she was wearing those sturdy lace-up Oxfords Marion needed for her arthritic feet. Dame Wendy was probably older than Marian was when I knew her, although at that time I thought she was ancient. I'm twenty years older now than she was when she died. Funny how one's perspectives change.

Marian was not like my own beautiful artistic mother. She talked to Hu about other people's motives. My gentle parents, at least in my company, discreetly voiced few opinions of others and unpleasant topics were not discussed.

Hu was nearly seven years older than me but my childhood too was in the early Thirties and my parents' financial struggles were kept from me, their only child. Then times improved for my family, while in southern Alberta, at Hu's home, times got worse. Veterinarian bills were not paid to his father who fell ill and died. No wonder a childhood friend tells me, "You had a sunny childhood."

I know I was civil to Marian, but it was an icy civility. And what that woman could have told me. Oh what stories. I could have said, *Marian, tell me about when you were in World War One as a nursing sister in Salonica. What was it like? Tell me about the soldier who carved the box on my bookshelf that's full of you and Tom's medals, and about the day you were on leave in Egypt, riding a camel, and the rider jouncing beside you was the handsome Welsh-Canadian veterinarian on leave from his horse battalion. He proposed marriage after not many more jounces, even though he had been married in Canada and had to get a divorce by act of Parliament. What did you think? You must have loved him very much. Like I love your son.*

Why didn't I say something like this? *And Marian, when the war ended, and you received your medal from the Prince of Wales, what was it like to come back to Peace River where your father, the former pastry cook from London, was trying to be the carrot king of the north? What did you think when you saw that big house of Tom's in the middle of downtown Calgary? How clever of you, after Tom's death, when Hu was fifteen, to turn the house into suites.*

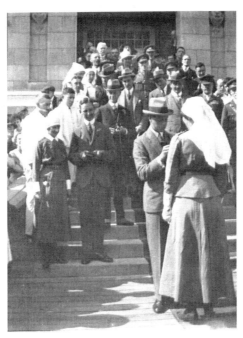

*Mother-in-law, Marian Osborne Harries, receiving medal from the
Duke of Windsor, in front of University Hospital, Edmonton — 1919*

Hu claims you're a good plain cook, and I remember you always had ginger ale mixed with Welch's grape juice with your dinners. My mother was perhaps a more adventuresome cook and oh how I was striving to become one, thanks to *The Joy of Cooking, Good Housekeeping, Ladies' Home Journal* and *Better Homes and Gardens. You sent your own bottled chicken to us in Edmonton. I'd never had that pinkish meat encased in sage flavored jelly. Though I know I must have written to thank you, again, I want you to know it was delicious. Why did I keep it a secret that I was secretly in awe of the way you quoted Shakespeare at the dinner table like Hu did And when our first child (named after your husband and son — Thomas Hu) was born, you knit him blue booties, sweater, hat and a tiny hot water bottle cover in seed and popcorn stitches, complete with tassels on everything. How you did this with your hand tremors, I'll never know. I'm glad you never knew about our little Tommy's death from polio a year after you died.*

One of those "If I had my life to life over, I would..." thoughts is: *try harder to understand and enjoy my mother-in-law.* But my very biggest regret, and it's a huge one, is that I never said: "Thanks Marian, for bearing and raising such a son as Hu."

To regret deeply is to live afresh. — Henry
David Thoreau, Journal, 1839

*This story can also be found in the Athabasca University's *Alberta Women's Memory Project* **under "memoir collection"**

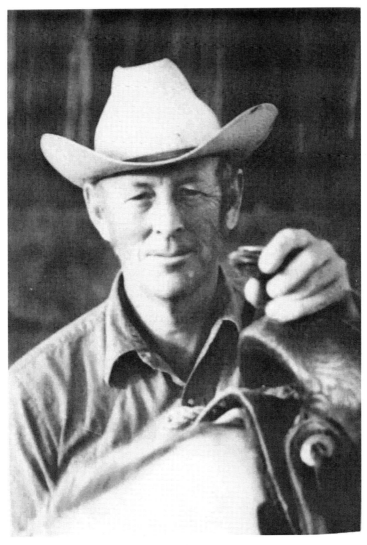

Hu

About Forget-Me-Nots

The teacher thanked me, the students clapped and some came over asking where they could buy my books since they knew my donated copies would be long-listed in their school library. One thirteen-year-old boy said, "I liked your stories, Mrs. Harries, and when you have your hundred-and-fifth birthday, I'll bring you forget-me-nots." After I'd thanked him profusely, and wiped away happy tears, Liam said, "I will, you know, 'cause I went on a hike last year with my parents and we came to a big patch of this flower and there weren't any houses around and my mother said they probably came up every year in this same spot. So I know where it is, and I'll bring you some."

This lovely late winter happening was after I'd read to a grade eight class from my book, *Girdles and Other Harnesses I Have Known.* In a story, "How I Want to Celebrate My 105th Birthday, If Cost is No Object," among things I hoped to do or see, were bouquets of flowers, including forget-me-nots.

> *Being naïve can be an adult's weakness, but*
> *a child's strength. — Anonymous*

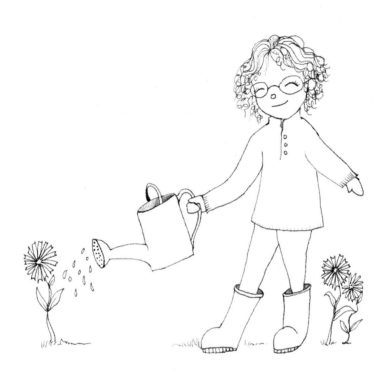

The End

Acknowledgements

Thanks for the encouragement to keep writing from my children and grandchildren and especially from my writing friends: Tuesday's Women's Collective Writing Group, Strathcona Senior's Thursday Critique Group and Friday's Creative Writing Group (where it all began). I am indebted to advice given at workshops provided by the Canadian Author's Association, Alberta Writer's Guild, Writer's Union, League of Canadian Poets and the Edmonton Stroll of Poets Society. I also want to thank Mary Dawe, Eunice Scarfe, Jack Bilsland and Shirley Serviss for early advice and Rachel Sentes, Laurie Greenwood, Farshad H. Niri, Margaret Macpherson, Marion Brooker and Ashley Patton for more recent advice. I am delighted by granddaughter Tasli Shaw's fine illustrations. and thank the Alberta Foundation for the Arts for making me think my work is worthwhile.

About the Author

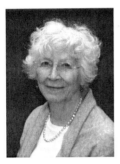

Joyce Harries was born an only child in 1928 in Edmonton, Alberta, Canada. She began writing humorous pieces about the vagaries of old age when she was almost seventy. Now, at eighty-four, her third book, *A Wise Old Girl's Own Almanac*, tells about turning twenty on her honeymoon and what she learned at the side of an academic, entrepreneurial, politician, rancher, Shakespeare-quoting husband.

They had six children together, losing their eldest son in the polio epidemic of 1953. She was a runway model from the age of fifteen until she was in her early forties. Joyce was widowed at fifty-eight, when husband Hu had a massive heart attack while riding his horse in a competition. She worked as a florist and caterer and ran artist's retreats at a vineyard in the Okanagan region of Canada.

She has had three books published: *Girdles and Other Harnesses I Have Known*, *Twice in a Blue Moon*, and *A Wise Old Girl's Own Almanac*. She has spouted poetry in cafés and became a guest speaker talking about the twists and turns in her world and the possibilities that await those who try something new in later life. People reading her books have gained insight through reflection on their own walk of life. She is presently working on a novel.

Why My Choice of Font

The reason I chose the Baskerville font was because it seems easier for old eyes to read than the more thinly inked, narrow-lined more modern fonts. I first was aware of Baskerville in two books published in Britain: *Miss Pettigrew Lives for a Day,* by Winifred Watson, published by Persephone Books Ltd. as a Persephone Book Classic, and *Mrs, Palfrey at the Claremont,* by Elizabeth Taylor, published by Virago Press Ltd. as a Virago Modern Classic.